AF891653

THE ADDICTION BLUEPRINT

The Holistic Guide to Understanding and Overcoming Addiction Today

addiction

/əˈdɪkʃn/

noun

- a chronic disease that involves a person losing control over a substance or behaviour, despite negative consequences.

blueprint

/ bluˈprɪnt/

noun

- a design or pattern that can be followed.

today

/təˈdeɪ/

Noun

- in this present time.

addiction blueprint today

/əˈdɪkʃn bluːˈprɪnt/təˈdeɪ/

- a design or structured understanding of how addiction develops, operates, and persists in this present time.

THE ADDICTION BLUEPRINT

The Holistic Guide to Understanding and Overcoming Addiction Today

Oliver Rolfe

Edited by David Moxon
MSc, BSc Hons (Psych), Cert Ed

Editorial advisor: Steps Together
Rehabilitation & Wellness

HH
BOOKS

Hammersmith Health Books
London, UK

This first edition is published by Hammersmith Health Books – an imprint of Hammersmith Books Limited
82 Wandsworth Bridge Road, London, SW6 2TF, UK
www.hammersmithbooks.co.uk

British Library Cataloguing in Publication Data: A CIP record of this book is available from the British Library.

Print ISBN 978-1-78161-270-5
Ebook ISBN 978-1-78161-271-2

Commissioning editor: Georgina Bentliff
Designed and typeset by: Julie Bennett of Bespoke Publishing Services
Cover design by: Madeline Meckiffe
Cover image: Yuliya Chsherbakova
Index: Jan Ross
Production: Anke Ueberberg
Printed and bound by: TJ Books, Padstow, Cornwall

CONTENTS

ABOUT THE AUTHOR

Oliver Rolfe is founder and CEO of Spartan International Group and focuses on life and career guidance and global investment banking recruitment. He studied accounting and finance and started his career with a leading global accounting firm. Oliver then sought a new challenge and moved into the executive search arena in 2003.

In 2003 he began his financial services recruitment career with a subsidiary of S3, one of the largest recruitment companies in Europe. Oliver has spent over 20 successful years specialising in mid- to senior-level individuals with outstanding track records in global equities.

In 2010, Oliver founded Spartan Partnership, and later Spartan International Executive Search, which is a global financial executive search firm. Oliver and Spartan remain focused on assisting those in the markets globally, both on the buy- and sell-sides of the business.

Oliver published his first book, *The Survivor's Guide to Your Career Today*, in 2019 and his second book, *The Holistic Guide To Your Health & Wellbeing Today*, in 2022, which achieved a notable ranking of #1 on Kobo and #2 on Amazon's Health & Wellbeing bestseller list. He has also been quoted in *The New York Times, Bloomberg, The Trade News, Gulf Times* and many more global publications.

His mission has always been to assist people in becoming the best they can possibly be.

ABOUT THE EDITOR

David Moxon MSc, BSc Hons (Psych), Cert Ed, has spent the last 30 years mentoring and educating people within the fields of health and psychology. He has been module leader for numerous degree programmes as well as supervising third-year dissertations.

As well as running a highly successful private consultancy, he has written three books: *Heinemann Themes in Psychology: Memory, Heinemann Themes in Psychology: Human Relationships,* and *Heinemann Psychology for AQA*. He has also edited a number of series within the field of psychology.

David retired from the academic world in 2020 and now runs a property company and is managing director of Head-a-Head, a specialist outplacement consultancy based in Mayfair. He had wanted to be involved in a book such as this for some time and thoroughly enjoyed the journey – as Oliver keeps on telling him: NOW is the time!

ABOUT STEPS TOGETHER REHABILITATION & WELLNESS

Steps Together Group is a trusted rehabilitation provider supporting adult individuals who suffer from a range of addiction problems as well as mental health, stress, and wellbeing challenges. Since its establishment in 2017, it has helped thousands of people and their families through a holistic, abstinent, client-centred, and multi-phase recovery programme. They facilitate medical detox across three of their sites. They understand that the longer a client spends in treatment, the better the chance of long-term recovery, as this gives clients time to delve further into their lives. The Group's independent semi-residential living offers long-term programmes in which clients learn to live in the community and have more responsibility for budgeting, shopping, cooking, looking for jobs, housing, and more family therapy before returning home. Guests remain part of the Steps Together family as they are offered free aftercare for 12 months and have the ability to continue therapy via their outpatient programme across all facilities in the UK. Their centres are located in Harley Street, Leicestershire, Nottinghamshire, and Merseyside.

Steps Together's programmes are structured across four distinct phases of treatment: clinical detox, intensive therapy programmes, second-stage independent living, outpatients, aftercare, and family support. Other services available to clients include flexible packages such as home detox, one-to-one therapy, and structured support programmes like 5-4-3-2-1 check-ins.

The organisation follows a holistic therapeutic model, combining clinical and wellness-based approaches. Treatments include cognitive behavioural therapy (CBT), dialectical behaviour therapy (DBT), psychotherapy, family therapy, and motivational interviewing, alongside complementary activities such as 12-step and SMART recovery groups, meditation, art and music therapy, fitness programmes, and holistic workshops. Steps Together also organises treatment around the '3 Rs' of recovery: Reset (detox and therapy), Reframe (developing new behaviours and lifestyle), and Recover (long-term stability).

Steps Together facilities are designed for comfort, recovery, and wellbeing. The Chestnuts in Leicestershire offers private and executive rooms, communal areas, therapy spaces, and a wellness room. George House in Nottinghamshire functions as both a residential and outpatient hub. Elizabeth House in Nottinghamshire provides semi-independent living with 13 en-suite rooms, communal lounges, and therapeutic areas. Rainford Hall and Fenny Bank Cottage in Merseyside extend services to that region. Most facilities feature peaceful gardens, home-cooked meals, and on-site staff supervision.

The team at Steps Together is highly experienced, combining professional qualifications with lived experience of recovery. Their psychiatry specialists include Dr Akif A Khan and Dr Aadil Shah, who bring expertise in addictions and general psychiatry. Therapy and rehabilitation services are led by John Wilson, Group Therapy Services Director, alongside a team of qualified therapists. The leadership team, including founder and CEO Darren Rolfe, Deputy CEO Steve Jones, and Operations Director Paul Mudie, provide strong oversight. Many staff members also contribute valuable peer support, having completed their own recovery journeys. All primary residential care services are regulated by the Care Quality Commission (CQC), ensuring safe and evidence-based practice. All centres are graded with a 'Good' outcome.

Admission begins with a free and confidential consultation to determine the most suitable programme. A full clinical assessment follows, and treatment plans are tailored to individual needs, ranging from seven to 84 nights, or longer. Detox programmes are carefully designed according to substance history and medical requirements, with each client receiving a personalised treatment plan.

The Steps Together Group also offers family interventions, which can be a loving way to support the family in getting a loved one into treatment (see Resources, page 499).

ACKNOWLEDGEMENTS

A huge thank you to David Moxon for working alongside me on this journey. Thank you to Darren Rolfe and Steps Together. I appreciate all you have done.

To my fantastic family, a wonderful and supportive wife, two beautiful children and our dog. Thank you for always trusting and believing in me. I love you all!

To all of you, thank you!

INTRODUCTION

In a comprehensive global health study conducted by the Institute for Health Metrics and Evaluation (IHME) in 2017 – as part of their flagship Global Burden of Disease Study – it was estimated that approximately 178 million people worldwide suffered from substance use disorders. Today, it is possible, if not probable, that this number has significantly increased.

- Alcohol use is responsible for around 107 million cases globally.
- Drug use accounts for approximately 71 million cases globally.

Addiction is characterised as a compulsive and repetitive disorder, defined by the persistent use of substances such as drugs or the continuous engagement in behaviours such as gambling, sexual activities, alcohol consumption, social media use, disordered eating (overeating, undereating, excess sugar consumption... etc.), prescription medication misuse, shopping, overworking, internet usage, video gaming, etc. These behaviours are pursued despite clear negative impacts on the individual's health, wellbeing, and relationships, often leading to significant harm to others. Public Health England sees addiction as a disease.

Addiction is one of the most complex and misunderstood challenges faced by individuals, families, and society alike. It weaves a tangled web of physical, emotional, and psychological dependency, often leaving those affected feeling trapped and isolated. What truly drives addiction? How does it take hold, and why do some people fall into its grip while others seem unaffected? This book explores these crucial questions, offering a comprehensive guide to understanding, recognising, and ultimately overcoming addiction.

The slippery slope towards addiction

Addiction exists on a sliding scale, with every individual positioned somewhere along it, because, by nature, humans are creatures of habit and routine. From small, everyday rituals like morning coffee or checking our phones, to more harmful behaviours, these habits are often our way of managing stress or emotions, or simply navigating the world. Our brains are wired to seek out patterns and predictability, so we naturally gravitate towards repetitive actions that provide comfort or reward. Over time, certain behaviours may become compulsive, driven by releases of the 'happy hormone' dopamine that reinforce the cycle, forming the basis for addiction. Recognising this connection is the first step towards addressing it. We must become aware of our habits, identifying which ones serve us and which are detrimental. Implementing mindful strategies, such as replacing harmful routines with healthier alternatives, and doing so consistently over time, can help break the cycle. It's about recognising the 'when' – understanding when a routine is tipping towards addiction and acting before it takes hold.

In our journey, we will dive into the 'how' and 'why' of addiction – how it starts, what fuels it, and why it persists. Addiction is more than just a bad habit or moral failing; it is deeply rooted in biology, psychology, and social context. The brain's reward system, emotional trauma, and environmental triggers often work together to create an overwhelming compulsion to seek solace in substances, behaviours, or activities that provide temporary relief but long-term damage.

Understanding the science behind addiction is key to understanding its grip. Why do certain individuals become addicted while others can walk away? What is it about some substances or behaviours that make them more addictive than others? This book delves into the brain's response to these stimuli, explaining why the connection between addiction and certain lifestyles, traumas, and genetic predispositions is so powerful.

Yet, beyond the 'why,' we must also address the 'what.' What can be done once addiction has taken root? Is there hope for recovery? The answer is a resounding yes. Through practical advice, proven strategies, and expert insights, this book aims to guide you through the recovery process. It explores when to seek help, the types of treatments available, and the essential steps needed to break free from the cycle of dependency.

Most importantly, this is not just a book about the problem of addiction - it is about solutions. Whether you are someone struggling with addiction yourself, a loved one trying to help, or simply seeking to understand this pervasive issue, you will find valuable insights and actionable steps to reclaim control, rebuild relationships, and create a future free from addiction's hold.

Addiction is not the end of the story. With the right understanding, tools, and timing, recovery is possible. Let this book be your guide on that journey.

Wholeness and addiction

The word 'Gestalt' is a German word that is notoriously difficult to translate into English. The closest equivalent might be 'wholeness' or 'completeness.' In the 1920s, a group of psychologists and philosophers adopted this term to reflect their understanding of human perception and behaviour. This group, known as the 'Gestaltists,' included Max Wertheimer (1880–1943), Kurt Koffka (1886–1941), and Wolfgang Köhler (1887–1967).

Rather than breaking down behaviours or problems into smaller parts, they advocated for understanding the whole, emphasising the idea that the sum of the parts does not necessarily explain the entirety of an experience.

A helpful analogy is to think of an old-fashioned TV screen made up of thousands of pixels. We could analyse each pixel individually – its colour, intensity, or placement – but it's only by stepping back and looking at the screen as a whole that we can recognise an image, a person, or an object. This principle is captured by the phrase: The whole is greater than the sum of its parts.

The Gestaltists' approach offered a different lens through which to view behaviour, and this idea is especially relevant when considering addiction. Much of modern science, particularly in areas like psychology, often focuses on isolating specific elements or behaviours. Addiction, however, is a complex and multifaceted issue, and breaking it down into its individual parts often misses the bigger picture. While detailed analysis – understanding triggers, environmental factors, and brain chemistry – is essential, we must also view addiction in the broader context of a person's life if we are to fully understand and address it.

So why start this book on addiction with this rather random philosophical idea?

Firstly, the concept of 'wholeness' can become somewhat lost in modern treatments for addiction, where attention is often given to isolated aspects of the issue – whether that's cravings, withdrawal symptoms, or patterns of relapse – rather than understanding the interconnectedness of all factors contributing to addiction. Society often encourages people to think in terms of specific problem areas.

Is your job stressing you out? Are you managing your relationships well? Are you sleeping enough? However, addiction rarely fits neatly into one category and is frequently a tangled web of physical, emotional, and psychological factors. To effectively combat it, we need to recognise the interplay between these areas rather than tackling each one in isolation.

Secondly, viewing addiction through the 'bigger picture' lens is essential to effective recovery. Breaking free from addiction isn't just about managing cravings or avoiding certain triggers – it's about understanding the whole of the person struggling with it. Achieving freedom from addiction requires recognising the interconnectedness of various dimensions of life: emotional health, physical wellbeing, social relationships, and psychological resilience.

Working through addiction requires a holistic approach. One's emotional state, mental health, and even energy levels can all impact recovery efforts. Recognising that these elements are deeply intertwined, just as the Gestaltists would suggest, is crucial for long-term success. Thinking of yourself as a whole person rather than as a collection of broken parts is key to recovery.

In the context of addiction, we are a system – a complex web of physical, mental, emotional, and environmental factors. Healing from addiction means addressing each of these dimensions together. Understanding that no single aspect operates in isolation helps reframe addiction as more than a collection of bad habits or poor choices. It is a manifestation of an imbalance in the whole system, and restoring balance requires seeing the whole picture.

In the words of Martin Luther King, Jr.: 'If you can't fly, run. If you can't run, walk. If you can't walk, crawl. No matter what, keep moving.' No matter where you are on your journey with addiction, recognising the bigger picture is a crucial step forward. Keep moving towards balance, even when progress feels slow.

IF NOT ME, THEN WHO?

My name is Oliver Rolfe. I am the Founder and CEO of Spartan International Group, an Executive Search Firm and Consultancy. So why have I written a book about addiction?

Before starting out on this book, I was already the author of two books – the first, *The Survivor's Guide To Your Career Today*, offering life and career guidance to young adults aged 16 to 25, related most obviously to my current career path; the second, *The Holistic Guide To Your Health & Wellbeing Today*, related more indirectly, aiming to help people in the financial services industry, and other professionals, make positive lasting change. Both books were inspired by my personal journey and a desire to help others with the knowledge I have gained along the way. So let me tell you more about my personal journey and how that has led me to writing *The Addiction Blueprint*.

My journey to Rainford Hall – A wellbeing reset

I never thought I would find myself needing help. I had never felt that I needed anyone else's help; I was doing pretty well on my own. Yet looking back now, I can see the signs had been there for a while – quietly present at first, then increasingly impossible to ignore.

It began with gentle concern from those closest to me. My family, in their caring and worried way, would ask, 'Are you okay?' or 'You look tired?' There were questions about my weight loss, why I seemed so drawn and hollow, and why I was drinking more. At the time, I brushed it all off. I thought I was coping. In reality, I was far from it.

Somewhere along the way, I had lost myself. I couldn't tell you what I enjoyed anymore or what made me feel alive. Every day felt like Groundhog Day. I was permanently tired, snappy, withdrawn. My mood was low, and I simply wasn't happy.

The month before everything unravelled, I had been travelling a lot. Jet lag, illness, fatigue – I was constantly running on empty. I kept thinking I just needed to get through the next day, the next task. Yet there was nothing left in the tank. I was running on fumes.

Then something shifted. My wife reached out to my brother. She knew I needed some help, even if I hadn't realised it yet. One afternoon, my brother and I went for a long walk – just the two of us. We spoke openly, something we hadn't done in a while. By the time we returned home, the decision had been made. I needed to take some time away to reset, to breathe, to find myself again. That afternoon, we sat down with my wife, and the three of us agreed: I would go to Rainford Hall for a Wellbeing Reset.

Getting there wasn't as straightforward as I had hoped. I remember scrolling through train websites, trying to figure out how to get from London to somewhere near Liverpool. There were no direct routes that day, and the thought of navigating connections was too much. My mind couldn't cope with the idea of switching platforms, managing timings, dragging bags. Eventually, I decided I would take a taxi straight to Rainford Hall. It seemed the simplest choice, and it gave me space to breathe before arriving.

The morning I left was quiet. The children had gone to school as usual. Just my wife and I remained. I packed my things, and we hugged, kissed, and said goodbye. There were a few shared tears.

I didn't know what was waiting for me – only that I had to go.

The three-and-a-half-hour drive that followed was largely uneventful, though strangely calming. The driver and I exchanged introductions and spoke briefly about the journey ahead. I felt the need to explain why someone might be taking a taxi all the way from London to Liverpool – not exactly an everyday occurrence. He listened without judgement, and after a short pause, shared a difficult situation he had recently gone through. There was an unspoken understanding between us. After that moment, we both seemed to recognise the value of silence. The rest of the journey passed quietly, save for a brief stop along the way. Hours later, as we turned off the main road and began navigating the long, winding drive, I caught my first glimpse of Rainford Hall. Nestled back among the trees, surrounded by sweeping grounds, it came into view like a quiet sanctuary. Something about it – the stillness, the setting – felt strangely comforting. I didn't know what was waiting for me inside; however, I knew that I was ready for it.

Walking into Rainford Hall for the first time, I was completely overwhelmed. I had no idea what to expect. I was nervous, anxious, on edge. Everything felt unfamiliar. Yet from the moment I arrived, the staff enveloped me with warmth and kindness. Their care was genuine. Their presence, reassuring. They made what felt like an alien experience somehow natural and human.

Within an hour of arrival, it was time for lunch. I remember walking into the dining area, head half down so as not to make eye contact with anyone, grabbing a small plate of food, and making my way to the furthest table there was from anyone. After about 30 seconds of me sitting down, a lovely staff member suggested that I sit with some of the other guests and placed me on another table. I found myself sitting down to lunch with two of the loveliest people – fellow guests, or as we affectionately called ourselves, 'the inmates'. Their openness and humour were a balm to my nerves. That first lunch felt like a step into something hopeful.

Later that afternoon, I took a walk through the grounds and called home. That simple act calmed me more than I can express. The setting was stunning - wild animals roamed freely, the trees stood tall and steady, the air was fresh and sweet with nature. It was, in a strange and unexpected way, a pleasure to be there. I felt like I could breathe.

That first night was strange. The room was quiet, unfamiliar. I lay there alone, listening to the subtle sounds of this new place. When I woke the next morning to birdsong - hundreds of tiny voices greeting the day - I felt oddly comforted. It was still early, long before my alarm, yet somehow it felt right. By night three, though, I did ask for some earplugs. I needed the extra hours of sleep!

The food at Rainford Hall was consistently brilliant. Every meal was fresh, nourishing and prepared with real care. The chefs weren't just talented - they were thoughtful. On my birthday, they went out of their way to create a feast for everyone, complete with a beautifully made cake. That sense of community, of being cared for, meant so much, especially on a day I would normally have spent with my family.

The group sessions were deeply moving. There were tears and laughter, often in equal measure. Listening to others share their stories - some full of pain, others laced with resilience - helped me to see that addiction and trauma are often deeply connected. It built a bond between us all. We became a family of sorts. Everyone had a role: there was a mum and dad, an uncle or grandfather figure, aunties and brothers and sisters. It was truly unique - a tribe of wounded souls helping each other heal. It was unlike anything I had experienced before.

Some of the best moments in the house were when everyone was all together at the end of the day in the main lounge. Some would watch TV together, usually a film or football match. Others would make bracelets, usually for others in the group. I still have mine! There would be board games in teams, pool tournaments, and the famous, or shall I say infamous, karaoke nights. We were told by staff that our group was a very close-knit community compared to others. I believe that we could all feel it and I am so grateful for those experiences and connections.

We often walked together through the surrounding countryside in the afternoons – through forests, across open fields. Wildlife was everywhere: hares darting, deer grazing, birds soaring, peacocks strutting. These walks became moments of calm, reflection and connection. Sometimes we talked deeply with staff who shared their own stories. Sometimes we simply walked in silence, side by side. Those walks reminded me of how powerful it is to just *be* – in nature, in motion, in the moment.

In fact, it was these walks that sparked something inside me – something I hadn't felt in a long time. Movement. Purpose. Those initial steps led to me completing the London Marathon in 2025. I fundraised for the National Association for Ankylosing Spondylitis, raising over £10,000. That journey started with one uncertain walk in the grounds of Rainford Hall.

Saying goodbye was harder than I expected. After all, I was desperate to be back with my family. Yet saying goodbye to people I had shared so much with was unexpectedly emotional. We had supported one another through raw, difficult moments. We had laughed, cried, and grown together. It wasn't just a programme. It was a community.

My time at Rainford Hall was more than a break. It was a beginning.

It gave me space to rest, to learn, and to reset. That time was invaluable – a turning point that allowed me to make real, lasting changes to my life.

Stepping out of the front door and back into 'the real world' felt surreal. On the train ride home, I read the notes and cards my fellow inmates had given me – messages of hope, humour, and love. A wave of emotion swept over me. Then I called my wife, told her I was on my way, and smiled. I was going home.

Coming home and seeing my family was an incredible feeling. I had missed them deeply – missed the simple joy of being together, of sharing space and laughter. It felt good to be back, to walk through the front door and know I was home.

Yet I knew I couldn't simply fall back into the same routine that had led me to burnout. This time, I chose to do things differently. I created a new rhythm – one that allowed me to be more present, more engaged, and far less consumed by the constant drive to work, need to do for others, and to provide. I began giving myself permission to slow down, to rest, to take care of myself – perhaps truly for the first time.

I stopped pushing myself relentlessly. I stopped chasing perfection or trying to be everything to everyone. I learned to be gentler with myself – to live in the moment rather than constantly preparing for the next.

Thanks to the support I received at Rainford Hall – both from the wonderful staff and from the friends I made there – returning to daily life felt manageable. The first week or so felt slightly unsteady, as all transitions do, although, I never felt alone. There were people to talk to, online groups where we could share progress, and of course, the unwavering support of my family and close friends. I felt that it was important to keep the individual therapy sessions going for some weeks after to ensure that I was fully on the right track and making the best decisions for me at that time.

That network - that community - became essential. It reminded me just how vital it is to stay connected. When you're isolated, old habits can creep back in. When you're surrounded by understanding and care, there's strength to move forward.

Healing is never a one-time fix. It's a process - a choice we make again and again, something to constantly work on. And for me, it began the moment I walked through the doors of Rainford Hall and chose to reset.

It was during this period of healing and reflection that the idea for this book began to take shape. As I pieced myself back together, I kept thinking: What would I have needed at the very beginning? What words, information, or guidance could have helped me understand what was happening before I hit the wall? Before the overworking, the exhaustion, the fatigue and numbness took over?

That question stayed with me, and more questions arose. There were questions from all directions. From the staff, from the teachings, from each other. Each time I would write down the question/s or topic/s to investigate later and learn more. So, I began to research and to write.

At first, it was a way to say thank you to my brother for his help, and, for myself - a way to process, to reflect, to untangle everything I had been through. As the words flowed, I realised this information might help others and that there was nothing of the sort available to buy. I reached out to Steps Together, the team that supported me through my reset, and shared my idea. They were encouraging from the very beginning and offered feedback on the themes and areas they believed would truly connect with others.

My publisher joined me a little later in the process. Their feedback was gentle yet honest, helping shape the book into something not only structured, readable, and useful, but also heartfelt. Through multiple drafts - some vulnerable, some painful, some cathartic - we created something I am proud of.

If a book like this had existed when I first began to struggle - back when I was tired all the time, irritable, lost in my own head - I think it would have helped me feel less alone and more connected. Maybe it would have helped me recognise the signs earlier. Maybe it would have helped me get help sooner.

My hope is that this book becomes exactly that for someone else. As the saying goes, 'sharing is caring.' I have found that to be true - the more you give, the more comes back to you. I hope by sharing my story, I can help someone else take that first step towards healing. Because you never know where that step might lead.

Whether you're right at the start of your journey, or somewhere in the messy middle, I want this to be a hand on your shoulder - a quiet voice reminding you that change is possible, and healing is real. You are not broken. You are not beyond help. And you don't have to go through it alone.

I have come to realise that personal awareness is just as vital as anything else we do for our wellbeing. It's the foundation for truly understanding our actions - what we're doing, why we're doing it, and whether it aligns with who we are. To know what's right for you, you must first know yourself. We are all unique, both in body and mind. No one else can ever fully understand your inner world, no matter how well-intentioned they may be. That insight must come from within.

Throughout this journey, and through much of the material explored in this book, I have deepened my understanding of the psychology behind addiction. More importantly, I have used that understanding to grow, heal, and better myself and my life. There is no single road to recovery, and certainly no such thing as perfection. However, there is progress, and that's what matters.

After actively applying many of the principles in this book to my own life, I have learned to pace myself. I have given myself permission to pause, to reflect, to rest - and yes, even to enjoy life. I still work as hard as I have ever done and remain involved in many projects, but do so with greater balance. I spend more time with my family, and I carve out space for myself, without the weight of guilt or pressure.

Throughout this book, I have woven my personal experiences into the general advice to highlight the deep, personal connection I have with each chapter and subject. These reflections are not just insights; they are moments from my own journey, shared to give context, meaning, and authenticity to the guidance offered.

Many of us strive to help others navigate the storms of life. However, I urge you to pay attention to your own warning signs, no matter how challenging they may be - because if you don't, you won't be there to help anyone else.

We never know when our time is up, but we can make the most of every moment. Life is fragile, and in an instant, everything can change. That's why it's crucial to seize the day and pursue your dreams with purpose.

Make your dreams and aspirations your reality.

PART I

UNDERSTANDING ADDICTION

What happens is not as important as how you react to what happens.

Ellen Glasgow, American novelist, 1873–1945

CHAPTER 1

WHY DID ADDICTION HAPPEN TO ME?

Addiction can feel like a deeply personal betrayal, as though your own body and mind have conspired against you. Understanding why addiction happened to you is a complex journey involving biological, psychological, and social factors. This chapter explores these dimensions, providing insight into why addiction might have taken hold, the connections that exist between various aspects of life and addiction, and how to address the problem effectively.

Understanding addiction: the basics

Addiction is a chronic condition characterised by the compulsive use of substances or engagement in behaviours despite adverse consequences. It's not merely a matter of willpower; it involves changes in the brain's structure and function that make it exceedingly difficult to control urges.

Biological factors: the brain's role

The brain plays a pivotal role in addiction. Neurotransmitters, the brain's chemical messengers, are significantly impacted by addictive substances. For instance, drugs like cocaine or alcohol can flood the brain with dopamine, a neurotransmitter associated with pleasure and reward. Over time, the brain's reward system becomes hijacked, requiring more of the substance to achieve the same effect, which can lead to addiction.

Genetics also contribute to susceptibility. Studies suggest that genetics can account for 40–60% of the risk of addiction. Certain genes may influence how your body metabolises substances or how you respond to them. For example, variations in the gene that codes for the enzyme alcohol dehydrogenase can affect how alcohol is processed, potentially influencing the likelihood of developing an alcohol-use disorder.

Psychological factors: the mind's influence

Addiction often stems from underlying psychological issues. Trauma, stress, and mental health disorders like anxiety or depression can increase vulnerability to addiction. Individuals may turn to substances as a way to cope with these conditions, seeking relief from pain or emotional turmoil. These connections are examined in detail in Chapters 11 to 21.

Cognitive factors also play a role. Those with certain personality traits, such as high impulsivity or risk-taking behaviours, may be more prone to addiction. Additionally, addiction can develop as a maladaptive coping mechanism. For example, someone who has experienced significant life stressors might use drugs or alcohol as a way to escape or numb their feelings.

Social factors: the impact of environment

The environment in which you live can significantly influence addiction risk. Social and environmental factors include:

- **Family history and dynamics:** Growing up in a family

where substance abuse is prevalent can normalise addictive behaviours. Familial patterns of addiction may also affect how one relates to substances.

- **Peer pressure and social circles:** Adolescents and young adults are particularly susceptible to peer influence. Being in a social circle where substance use is common can increase the likelihood of developing similar habits.
- **Socio-economic status:** Financial instability and associated stressors can heighten vulnerability to addiction. Individuals in challenging socio-economic situations may use substances as a form of escape or as a means to cope with daily struggles.

These connections are examined in detail in Chapters 22 to 38.

The connection between factors

Addiction often results from a complex interplay of these biological, psychological, and social factors. For instance, a person with a genetic predisposition to addiction who experiences significant stress or trauma may be more likely to develop an addiction than someone who lacks these combined risk factors.

The interaction between these factors means that addressing addiction requires a multifaceted approach. Understanding how these elements interconnect can help in formulating a comprehensive plan for recovery.

What to do: taking the first steps

If you find yourself struggling with addiction, there are steps you can take to address it:

1. **Acknowledge the problem:** Recognising that you have

an addiction is the first and crucial step towards recovery. Denial can prevent you from seeking the help you need.

2. **Building healthy habits:** Addiction often leads to the breakdown of healthy routines and habits. Part of recovery involves re-establishing a balanced lifestyle, including proper nutrition, regular exercise, and adequate sleep. These habits not only help the body recover but also improve mental wellbeing, reducing the risk of relapse.

3. **Seek professional help:** Addiction often requires professional intervention. Consulting with a healthcare provider, addiction specialist, or therapist can provide you with a tailored treatment plan. Options include cognitive behavioural therapy (CBT), medication-assisted treatment, and support groups.

4. **Build a support network:** Surround yourself with supportive individuals who understand your journey. Support groups, family, and friends can provide encouragement and accountability.

5. **Develop coping strategies:** Work with a therapist to develop healthy coping mechanisms for dealing with stress and emotional pain. This might include mindfulness practices, exercise, or engaging in hobbies.

6. **Set realistic goals:** Recovery is a process that takes time. Set achievable goals for yourself and celebrate small victories along the way.

When to seek help

The right time to seek help is as soon as you recognise that addiction is impacting your life. Waiting until the consequences become severe can make recovery more challenging. Early intervention can lead to more effective treatment and a better chance at long-term recovery.

My personal experience

There came a period when I felt like something was out of sync, and the energy that had once driven me started to wane. I kept going, telling myself I was simply tired, although it was far deeper than that. The long hours, constant striving, and inability to pause had left my body depleted and my mind frayed. I began waking up feeling no more rested than when I had gone to bed, and my thoughts moved in circles I couldn't break free from. I didn't understand the full weight of what was happening at the time. My body was speaking through exhaustion, and my spirit was asking for stillness. It felt as though I had been moving further away from myself, until I could no longer ignore the signals. That deep weariness became the turning point - a silent invitation to stop, reflect, and make space for something more sustainable. It was not about failure, it was about reaching a point where something had to change.

Conclusion

Understanding why addiction happened to you - or someone you care for - involves exploring a range of biological, psychological, and social factors. By acknowledging these elements and taking proactive steps towards recovery, you can begin to reclaim control over your life. Remember, addiction is not a personal failure; it is a complex condition that requires compassion and a well-rounded approach to overcome. Seeking help is a sign of strength, and taking the steps outlined in this chapter can set you on the path towards a healthier and more fulfilling life.

CHAPTER 2

BREAKING THE STIGMA OF ADDICTION

Addiction is often misunderstood, not just as a personal failing but as a moral weakness. These misconceptions fuel stigma, one of the most significant barriers preventing individuals from seeking the help they desperately need. In this chapter, we explore the relationship between addiction and stigma, how stigma manifests, why it hinders people from reaching out for support, and what can be done to combat it.

What stigma is

Stigma is a set of negative beliefs and attitudes that society or individuals hold towards a particular group of people. In the context of addiction, stigma manifests in assumptions that those struggling with substance use disorders (SUDs) or other addictions, are weak, irresponsible, or even dangerous. This judgement is often compounded by societal norms that equate self-control with moral virtue, implying that those who become addicted have chosen their path or lack the discipline to stop.

Stigma is both societal and internalised. External stigma comes from family members, friends, colleagues, and the wider public, while internalised stigma is when the individual battling addiction starts to believe these negative stereotypes about themselves.

How stigma prevents people from seeking help

Stigma plays a significant role in discouraging individuals from seeking help for several reasons. Understanding how this works requires us to consider several factors that reinforce stigma and its consequences.

1. **Fear of judgement and discrimination:** One of the most powerful deterrents created by stigma is the fear of judgement and discrimination. Those battling addiction often anticipate being viewed as failures, criminals, or socially deviant. The possibility of being ostracised by family, rejected by employers, or dismissed by medical professionals leads many to suffer in silence. A person might be unwilling to admit they have a problem because they fear losing their job, being rejected by friends, or experiencing strained family relationships. The desire to avoid judgement overrides the impulse to seek help, trapping individuals in cycles of shame and secrecy.

2. **Shame and self-blame:** When stigma is internalised, it can lead to feelings of shame, guilt, and self-blame. Individuals begin to see themselves as flawed or unworthy of support. The very nature of addiction already fosters cycles of guilt - the inability to stop despite recognising the harm being done. Stigma amplifies this guilt, creating a psychological burden that makes it difficult for individuals to believe they deserve help.

3. **Shame fosters isolation:** A person who feels ashamed of their addiction may withdraw from loved ones, avoiding

opportunities where they might be encouraged to seek help. Without social support, the addiction worsens, and the cycle becomes harder to break.

4. **Misinformation and myths:** Stigma is often underpinned by widespread myths and misconceptions about addiction. For example, many people still believe addiction is a choice or a sign of weak willpower. These false beliefs feed into the shame felt by individuals and the discrimination they face from others. These myths also exist in the healthcare system. Some healthcare providers may unconsciously treat people with addiction differently, assuming that they are less motivated or less compliant with treatment. This medical stigma can result in inadequate care, making it even more difficult for someone to get the help they need.

5. **Legal and social consequences:** In many societies, the legal framework around drug use adds another layer of stigma. In the UK, while possession of drugs is illegal, addiction is a recognised medical condition. However, the criminalisation of drug use means that individuals risk legal penalties if they admit to substance abuse, creating another barrier to seeking help. Even if they avoid legal consequences, those with a history of addiction may be viewed as untrustworthy or risky in their personal and professional lives, reinforcing the reluctance to come forward.

Why does stigma persist?

Stigma around addiction persists because it is deeply rooted in long-standing societal beliefs about morality, health, and self-control. Several factors contribute to its endurance:

1. **Lack of education:** Many people do not understand the complexity of addiction as a medical condition. Addiction is often seen as a moral failing, despite overwhelming evidence that it is a chronic illness involving neurological changes and a complex interplay of genetic, psychological, and environmental factors.

2. **Fear and misunderstanding:** Addiction is often associated with antisocial behaviour, criminality, and danger, which leads to fear. This fear perpetuates stigma, as society views addiction as something to be punished rather than treated. When addiction is portrayed as dangerous or corrupting, people avoid engaging with it in any meaningful way, preferring to keep their distance from those struggling with it.

3. **Media representation:** The media play a crucial role in shaping perceptions of addiction. Sensationalist reporting that focuses on extreme cases of addiction, such as overdose deaths or violent crimes, can skew public understanding. Rarely do we see media coverage of people in recovery or stories that frame addiction as a treatable illness. Instead, negative portrayals reinforce harmful stereotypes.

4. **Cultural values of self-sufficiency:** In many Western societies, the idea of self-sufficiency and individualism is highly valued. Asking for help can be seen as a sign of weakness. This cultural belief feeds into the stigma surrounding addiction, as those who cannot 'pull themselves together' are viewed with disdain. The pressure to maintain the appearance of control and self-reliance can prevent people from admitting that they need help.

How to combat stigma

While stigma is deeply entrenched, there are steps that individuals and society can take to combat it, thereby creating a more supportive environment for those struggling with addiction.

1. **Education and awareness:** Raising public awareness about the true nature of addiction is one of the most effective ways to reduce stigma. Public health campaigns that highlight addiction as a medical condition, explain the science behind it, and showcase recovery stories can challenge misconceptions. It's crucial that people understand that addiction is treatable, and recovery is possible. We can all do our bit to encourage schools, workplaces, and healthcare systems to incorporate education about addiction and mental health to reduce stigma and encourage early intervention. The more informed people are, the less likely they are to perpetuate harmful stereotypes.

2. **Changing the narrative:** The language we use around addiction matters. Terms like 'junkie' or 'addict' are dehumanising and contribute to stigma. Instead, using 'person-first' language (e.g., 'a person with a substance use disorder') humanises the individual and focuses on the condition rather than defining the person by their illness. Shifting the way we talk about addiction can reshape societal perceptions.

3. **Supporting recovery stories:** Sharing stories of individuals who have sought treatment and are in recovery can inspire others and reduce the shame associated with addiction. Recovery stories highlight the fact that people can and do recover from addiction, breaking the stereotype that addiction is a hopeless condition. Support groups, podcasts, and documentaries featuring real-life experiences can provide hope and foster understanding.

4. **Peer support and advocacy:** Encouraging peer-led initiatives where individuals who have been through recovery support others can be immensely powerful. Peer advocates can help to de-stigmatise addiction by normalising the process of seeking help. Their unique insight allows them to challenge stigma both from a societal and an individual perspective, creating safe spaces for others to come forward.

5. **Policy change:** We can all help to encourage government and institutions to adopt policies that treat addiction as a public health issue, not a criminal one. Decriminalisation of drug use and ensuring that medical treatment is accessible without fear of legal reprisal are key steps in reducing stigma. Policies that offer protection for employees in recovery can encourage more people to seek treatment without the fear of losing their livelihoods.

When to seek help

Breaking through the barrier of stigma is never easy, however, there are moments when seeking help becomes critical. If you are struggling with addiction, remember that the longer you wait, the harder it becomes to address the problem. The best time to seek help is always now – before the addiction deepens its grip, before relationships are further damaged, and before health deteriorates further.

Those in a position to help – family members, friends, employers, and healthcare providers – need to be vigilant and compassionate. Encouraging someone to seek help early can prevent the downward spiral that stigma often fuels.

Conclusion

Stigma is a powerful force in perpetuating addiction and preventing people from seeking help. It thrives on misinformation, fear, and societal values that equate addiction with moral failure. However, by raising awareness, changing the narrative, and supporting policy change, we can dismantle the stigma around addiction. In doing so, we create a society where individuals feel empowered to seek the help they need, without fear of judgement or rejection.

The path to recovery is difficult enough without the added burden of stigma. By addressing stigma head-on, we can remove one of the greatest barriers to treatment and give those struggling with addiction the chance to reclaim their lives.

CHAPTER 3

THE WHY, HOW, WHAT, AND WHEN OF ADDICTION

Addiction is often misunderstood, misrepresented, and unfairly stigmatised, as we have seen. However, it is, at its core, a deeply human experience - an intricate dance between our psychology, environment, and biology. The connection with addiction is not a straightforward cause-and-effect relationship; it is shaped by a complex web of interrelated factors as this book goes on to highlight.

Understanding these connections is key to preventing, addressing, and ultimately healing addiction. In this chapter, we take an initial, overall look at the connections that lead to addiction - why it happens, how it happens, what makes it so powerful, and what can be done to break free from its grip. In Chapter 6 we explore this interconnectedness further.

The biology of addiction: why it happens

At a biological level, addiction fundamentally alters the brain's reward system. The human brain is hardwired to seek pleasure and avoid pain. This is part of our survival instinct; food, social connections, and even sexual activity release chemicals, especially dopamine, which make us feel good and motivate us to continue these behaviours.

Substances like drugs and alcohol, or behaviours like gambling and compulsive internet use, hijack this reward system. They flood the brain with an excessive amount of dopamine, far more than natural rewards like food or socialising. Over time, the brain begins to crave this intense stimulation, and normal pleasures no longer satisfy in the same way. This leads to a vicious cycle where the person feels compelled to seek out the addictive substance or behaviour to feel 'normal.' As tolerance builds, they need increasing amounts to achieve the same effect, deepening the dependency.

The psychological and emotional drivers: how it happens

Psychological factors also play a significant role in addiction. People often turn to addictive substances or behaviours as a way to cope with emotional pain, stress, anxiety, or trauma. Addiction, in this sense, is frequently a maladaptive coping mechanism - an attempt to escape or numb overwhelming emotions.

The relationship between addiction and mental health disorders such as depression (Chapter 20), anxiety (Chapter 21), and post-traumatic stress disorder (PTSD) (Chapter 26) is well-documented. Many individuals struggling with addiction have underlying emotional distress or unresolved trauma. In some cases, people develop addiction as a way to self-medicate, seeking relief from the symptoms of these mental health issues. However, this temporary relief can lead to a deeper sense of isolation, shame, and self-loathing, perpetuating the cycle of addiction.

Environmental and social influences: what makes it happen

Addiction rarely occurs in isolation. Environmental and social factors heavily influence its development as already described. (Part II(b) of this book then goes on to look at these many factors in detail.) These include family dynamics (Chapter 28), peer pressure, socio-economic status (Chapter 24), exposure to addictive substances (Chapter 22), and even cultural attitudes toward addiction.

Growing up in an environment where addiction is normalised or where emotional support is lacking can increase the likelihood of developing addictive behaviours. Children raised in households where a parent is addicted may learn these behaviours and repeat the cycle. Similarly, those who face chronic stress - whether from financial hardship, social instability, or lack of community - may be more susceptible to addiction as a form of escape (see Chapter 25).

Peers also exert considerable influence. Adolescence and early adulthood, times of identity formation and social development, are periods when people are particularly vulnerable to peer pressure. Social circles that encourage drug use, excessive drinking, or other high-risk behaviours can lead individuals down the path of addiction. The need to fit in, to be accepted, or to belong can make individuals willing to take risks they otherwise wouldn't.

The neurological connection: why the brain gets hooked

It is important to understand that addiction is not simply about willpower or a lack of moral fibre. The neurological changes that take place during addiction make it extremely difficult for people to simply 'quit'. The brain undergoes structural changes that reinforce the addictive behaviour, creating a powerful feedback loop that overrides rational decision-making.

The prefrontal cortex, the part of the brain responsible for judgement, self-control, and decision-making, becomes impaired as addiction develops. This can result in impaired judgement, making it harder for individuals to recognise the negative consequences of their actions. The brain's reward system, driven by the release of dopamine, also becomes rewired to prioritise the addictive substance or behaviour over all else, even when it is causing harm.

These changes can persist long after a person stops using the substance or engaging in the behaviour, which is why recovery is often a lifelong process. Cravings can resurface even years after someone has 'quit,' triggered by stress, exposure to the substance, or even certain emotional states. This neurological component underscores why addiction is considered a chronic condition, similar to other chronic diseases such as diabetes or heart disease. (See Chapter 10 on relapse in addiction.)

What to do: breaking the cycle of addiction

The road to recovery from addiction (see Part III) is challenging but not impossible. It begins with recognising the problem and understanding that addiction is not a failure of character but rather a condition that requires treatment. The first step is to acknowledge the connection with addiction and seek help. This could be through professional therapy, rehabilitation programmes, support groups, or a combination of these approaches.

Treatment often involves addressing both the physical and psychological aspects of addiction. Medications can sometimes help to manage withdrawal symptoms and reduce cravings. However, talking therapy plays a critical role in helping individuals understand the underlying emotional and psychological drivers of their addiction.

Cognitive behavioural therapy (CBT), for example, can help individuals identify and change the thought patterns and behaviours that contribute to their addiction. Psychotherapy may be used to work through trauma, depression, or anxiety that might be fuelling the addictive behaviour. Group therapy or support groups, such as Alcoholics Anonymous (AA) or Narcotics Anonymous (NA), can provide valuable community support and accountability, helping people realise they are not alone in their struggle.

When to take action

There is no 'perfect' time to seek help for addiction; the most important thing is to take action as soon as the problem is recognised. Addiction is progressive - it tends to worsen over time, leading to increased physical, emotional, and social harm. Therefore, early intervention is crucial. The sooner someone seeks help, the easier it is to reverse the damage and begin the healing process.

That said, it is never too late to seek help, no matter how deep the addiction has become. Recovery is always possible with the right support and treatment. It's important to realise that recovery is not a one-time event but an ongoing process that requires effort, patience, and resilience.

Why the connection matters

Understanding the interconnectedness of addiction is vital for both prevention and treatment. It highlights that addiction is not a matter of weak willpower; it is a multifaceted condition involving biological, psychological, and social factors. Recognising this connection shifts the conversation from blame and shame to compassion and treatment, opening the door to effective support and recovery.

This connection also underscores the importance of addressing the root causes of addiction. By tackling issues like trauma, mental health, social inequality, and environmental stress, we can prevent addiction from taking hold in the first place. Prevention efforts that focus on building resilience, providing support, and fostering healthy environments can significantly reduce the risk of addiction in vulnerable populations.

My personal experience

My experiences through overworking and burnout taught me that what I was facing was not simply a habit or a moment of weakness; it was a complex interplay of emotions, behaviours, and physical responses shaped over time. The exhaustion and overworking had created patterns that affected every part of my life. Recognising the many layers involved made me see why a full reset was needed to address all aspects of wellbeing, not just surface symptoms. It was by understanding the layers beneath and bringing them to the surface that set me on the right path.

Conclusion

Addiction is a complex and deeply personal experience, but it is not an insurmountable one. By understanding the connections – why it happens, how it happens, and what makes it so difficult to escape – we can begin to break down the stigma surrounding addiction and open the door to recovery. The key to overcoming addiction lies in addressing the underlying factors that contribute to it, seeking help, and committing to a path of healing and self-discovery.

Whether you or someone you know is grappling with addiction, it is essential to remember that recovery is possible. The connections that bind us to addiction can be untangled, and a life of freedom and fulfilment awaits on the other side.

CHAPTER 4

THE FIVE CHARACTERISTICS OF ADDICTION

Addiction is a profound and often perplexing condition that affects many aspects of an individual's life. To better understand addiction and its impact, it is crucial to explore its defining characteristics. This chapter delves into five key characteristics of addiction: tolerance, withdrawal, denial/rationalisation, loss of willpower, and preoccupation. It examines how each characteristic manifests, why each occurs, and effective strategies for addressing them.

1. Tolerance

What it is: Tolerance refers to the need for increasing amounts of a substance or behaviour to achieve the desired effect. Over time, the initial dose or behaviour becomes less effective, leading individuals to consume or engage more to experience the same level of satisfaction or relief.

How it happens: Tolerance develops as the body and brain adapt to the repeated presence of the substance or behaviour. This adaptation often involves physiological changes, such as alterations in neurotransmitter levels or receptor sensitivity, which diminish the substance's effects over time.

Why it matters: Understanding tolerance is essential as it highlights the progressive nature of addiction. It explains why individuals often escalate their usage or engagement, increasing their risk of further harm and complicating the recovery process.

What to do: Managing tolerance typically involves a period of abstinence or reduction in use, allowing the body to reset and regain sensitivity. Medical supervision may be necessary, particularly if the substance or behaviour has led to significant physiological dependence. Therapeutic interventions can help address the psychological aspects of tolerance.

When to act: Action should be taken when there is a noticeable increase in the amount or frequency of the substance or behaviour required to achieve the same effect. This often signifies the development of tolerance and the need for professional help to manage it effectively.

2. Withdrawal

What it is: Withdrawal encompasses a range of physical and psychological symptoms that occur when the substance or behaviour is reduced or discontinued. Symptoms can vary widely, from mild discomfort to severe distress, depending on the substance or behaviour involved.

How it happens: Withdrawal occurs because the body and brain have become reliant on the substance or behaviour to function normally. When it is removed, the brain must readjust to its absence, leading to an imbalance in neurotransmitters and other physiological processes.

Why it matters: Recognising withdrawal is critical for understanding the challenges faced during the recovery process. It highlights the physical and psychological hurdles that need to be addressed to support successful recovery.

What to do: Withdrawal should be managed under medical supervision, especially if symptoms are severe or even potentially life-threatening. A structured detoxification programme, combined with psychological support, can help ease the transition and minimise discomfort.

When to act: Professional help should be sought when withdrawal symptoms become apparent or if they pose significant risks to health. Early intervention can help mitigate the effects and support a smoother recovery process.

3. Denial/rationalisation

What it is: Denial and rationalisation involve a refusal to acknowledge the severity of the addiction or the impact it has on one's life. Denial involves rejecting the reality of the problem, while rationalisation involves justifying or excusing the behaviour.

How it happens: These mechanisms often stem from a desire to avoid facing the negative consequences of addiction. They provide temporary relief from guilt or shame but ultimately prevent individuals from seeking necessary help or making meaningful changes.

Why it matters: Understanding denial and rationalisation is vital because they hinder the recognition of addiction as a serious issue. They can delay intervention and treatment, exacerbating the addiction and its consequences.

What to do: Addressing denial and rationalisation requires a compassionate approach that encourages self-reflection and honesty. Therapy, particularly cognitive behavioural therapy (CBT), can help individuals confront their beliefs and attitudes towards their addiction, fostering acceptance and readiness for change.

When to act: Interventions should be considered when there is a persistent pattern of denying or rationalising addictive behaviours. Early engagement in therapy or support groups can facilitate awareness and encourage acceptance of the addiction.

4. Loss of willpower

What it is: Loss of willpower refers to the diminished ability to resist the urge to engage in the addictive behaviour or consume the substance. This characteristic reflects the struggle to control impulses and make rational decisions in the face of addiction.

How it happens: The brain's reward system becomes compromised in addiction, making it increasingly difficult to exert self-control. Neurochemical changes reduce the effectiveness of willpower, leading individuals to act against their better judgement.

Why it matters: Recognising loss of willpower is crucial for understanding why addiction can be so overpowering. It underscores the need for external support and strategies to bolster self-control and decision-making.

What to do: Strategies to combat loss of willpower include developing a structured plan for behaviour change, employing coping mechanisms, and seeking support from therapy and support groups. Building a strong support network and setting clear, achievable goals can also help to enhance willpower.

When to act: Action should be taken when the inability to control impulses becomes evident and starts to interfere with daily functioning or relationships. Professional support and structured programmes can help in regaining self-control and making positive changes.

5. Preoccupation

What it is: Preoccupation involves an intense focus on the substance or behaviour, where it dominates thoughts and activities. This characteristic reflects how addiction can overshadow other aspects of life, consuming significant mental and emotional energy.

How it happens: Preoccupation arises because the brain's reward system becomes overly fixated on the substance or behaviour, leading to persistent thoughts, cravings, and planning around it. This focus displaces other interests and responsibilities.

Why it matters: Understanding preoccupation highlights how addiction can become the central focus of an individual's life. It underscores the need for strategies that address not only the behaviour but also the cognitive and emotional patterns associated with addiction.

What to do: Managing preoccupation involves creating a balanced life with engaging activities and responsibilities that shift focus away from the addiction. Talking therapy, particularly approaches like mindfulness and cognitive restructuring, can help individuals reframe their thoughts and reduce obsessive focus.

When to act: Intervention should be considered when preoccupation with the addictive behaviour or substance starts to dominate an individual's thoughts and activities, leading to neglect of other areas of life. Support from therapy and structured activities can help redirect focus and rebuild a more balanced life.

Conclusion

Recognising and understanding the five characteristics of addiction - tolerance, withdrawal, denial/rationalisation, loss of willpower, and preoccupation - provides a comprehensive view of how addiction manifests and impacts individuals. Addressing each characteristic through targeted strategies and seeking appropriate support can significantly enhance the chances of recovery and improve overall quality of life.

CHAPTER 5

THE FOUR Cs OF ADDICTION

Addiction is a complex and multifaceted issue, often characterised by the 'four Cs': craving, control, consequences, and compulsion. Understanding these core elements can provide valuable insights into the nature of addiction and guide effective intervention strategies.

1. Craving

What it is: Craving refers to an intense and often overwhelming desire to engage in a behaviour or consume a substance, despite recognising the potential for negative outcomes. It is a powerful force that drives individuals to seek out their addiction, whether it be alcohol, drugs, gambling, or other compulsive behaviours.

How it happens: Cravings are rooted in the brain's reward system. When an individual engages in addictive behaviour, the brain releases neurotransmitters like dopamine, which create feelings of pleasure and reinforcement. Over time, the brain becomes conditioned to associate the substance or behaviour with these rewarding feelings, leading to persistent cravings.

What to do: Effective management of cravings involves several strategies:

- **Awareness and mindfulness:** Recognising and acknowledging cravings without immediately succumbing to them can help individuals regain control. Mindfulness practices can increase awareness and help manage the emotional responses associated with cravings.
- **Distraction techniques:** Engaging in alternative activities or hobbies can divert attention away from cravings. Exercise, creative pursuits, and social interactions can serve as effective distractions.
- **Support systems:** Building a strong network of friends, family, or support groups can provide emotional support and practical advice, helping individuals navigate their cravings more effectively.

2. Control

What it is: Control refers to the ability of an individual to regulate their behaviour and resist the urge to engage in addictive activities. The loss of control is a hallmark of addiction, where individuals find themselves unable to limit their consumption or behaviour despite adverse consequences.

How it happens: Addiction often disrupts normal brain function, impairing the ability to exercise self-control. The brain's reward system becomes hijacked by the substance or behaviour, making it difficult to override impulses. Additionally, psychological factors such as stress, trauma, and emotional dysregulation can further erode control.

What to do: Regaining control involves:

- **Setting boundaries:** Establishing clear limits on behaviour and consumption can provide structure and help in managing addiction.

- **Therapeutic interventions:** Cognitive behavioural therapy (CBT) and other therapeutic approaches can help individuals understand and modify their thought patterns and behaviours, enhancing self-control.
- **Developing coping skills:** Learning and practising coping strategies for stress and emotional challenges can reduce reliance on addictive behaviours.

3. Consequences

What they are: Consequences are the negative outcomes and impacts resulting from addictive behaviours. These can range from physical health issues, such as liver disease or cardiovascular problems, to social and psychological effects, such as strained relationships or diminished self-esteem.

Why they matter: Understanding and acknowledging the consequences of addiction is crucial for motivating change. The pain and difficulty associated with consequences can serve as a powerful impetus for seeking help and making behavioural changes. Additionally, recognising the broader impact of addiction on one's life can foster a sense of urgency and commitment to recovery.

What to do: Addressing consequences involves:

- **Seeking professional help:** Engaging with healthcare professionals, such as doctors or addiction specialists, can provide necessary medical care and support for managing and mitigating consequences.
- **Rebuilding relationships:** Repairing damaged relationships and rebuilding trust with loved ones can be an essential part of recovery. Open communication and taking responsibility for past actions are key components.
- **Implementing lifestyle changes:** Adopting healthier

lifestyle habits, including proper nutrition, exercise, and stress management, can help reverse some of the negative effects of addiction and improve overall wellbeing.

4. Compulsion

What it is: 'Compulsion' refers to the uncontrollable urge to repeat an addictive behaviour despite the desire to stop. It is characterised by a persistent drive to engage in the behaviour, often accompanied by a sense of powerlessness or inevitability.

How it happens: Compulsive behaviour is often driven by the brain's altered reward circuitry, which has become accustomed to the highs associated with the addictive substance or behaviour. This alteration creates a cycle where the compulsion to engage in the behaviour becomes a predominant force, overriding rational thought and self-control.

What to do: Managing compulsion involves:

- **Professional treatment:** Therapy, including behavioural therapies and pharmacological treatments, can address the underlying neurological and psychological factors contributing to compulsive behaviour.
- **Support networks:** Engaging with support groups and counselling can provide accountability and emotional support, helping individuals navigate their compulsions.
- **Lifestyle adjustments:** Making changes to one's environment and daily routines to minimise triggers and stressors can reduce the likelihood of compulsive behaviour.

Conclusion

The four Cs of addiction - craving, control, consequences, and compulsion - provide a framework for understanding the complexities of addiction. By exploring these elements, individuals and practitioners can develop more effective strategies for managing and overcoming addiction. Recognising the interplay between these factors is essential for developing a comprehensive approach to treatment and recovery. Through awareness, intervention, and support, it is possible to break the cycle of addiction and achieve lasting change.

CHAPTER 6

THE INTERCONNECTED WEB OF ADDICTION

As we will see throughout this book, addiction is rarely a standalone issue. It usually intertwines with other facets of our lives, impacting not only us/the individual but also our relationships, health, and society. At the heart of addiction lies a deeper connection with five key elements: disease, disconnection, dishonesty, distraction, and detachment. Understanding these connections can illuminate the path to recovery and provide insight into why addiction takes hold and persists.

In this chapter, we explore the intricate relationships between addiction and these five elements. We uncover why these connections exist, how they manifest, and what actions can be taken to address them.

1. Addiction and disease

Addiction has a profound connection with disease, as both a cause and an effect. Addiction itself is often classified as a chronic disease, affecting the brain's structure and function, while also leading to or exacerbating physical and mental health conditions. Chapter 11 looks at this in greater detail, but this section introduces the key concepts.

How addiction leads to disease

Addictive substances and behaviours directly impact the body. For example, alcohol and drug addiction can lead to liver disease, heart conditions, respiratory issues, and weakened immune function. Addiction also manifests in mental health disorders, such as depression, anxiety, and stress-related illnesses.

This connection is particularly evident in the way addiction rewires the brain. The repeated exposure to addictive substances or behaviours alters the brain's reward system, causing a surge of dopamine that eventually results in tolerance. Over time, this imbalance contributes to a range of health issues, marking addiction as both a physical and mental disease.

Why this happens

The relationship between addiction and disease is cyclical. Mental health issues such as depression or anxiety can drive individuals to seek relief in addictive substances or behaviours, while addiction, in turn, worsens these conditions. Physical ailments can also lead to addiction, particularly when people become reliant on painkillers or other substances to manage chronic pain.

What to do

Effective addiction treatment requires addressing both the addiction and the associated health conditions. Integrating physical and mental healthcare into addiction recovery programmes is essential for breaking the cycle of disease and addiction. Seeking professional help early can prevent the progression of both addiction and related illnesses.

2. Addiction and disconnection

Disconnection, whether from society, relationships, or oneself, plays a pivotal role in addiction. Many individuals struggling with addiction report feelings of loneliness and isolation, and a sense of not belonging. This sense of separation fuels the addiction, which in turn deepens the disconnection.

How disconnection fuels addiction

Disconnection leaves a void that many people attempt to fill with substances or compulsive behaviours. Addiction often becomes a coping mechanism, an attempt to soothe the emotional pain caused by a lack of connection to others or a fractured relationship with oneself. For example, people may turn to alcohol or drugs to escape feelings of loneliness or a lack of purpose.

Once addiction takes hold, it further isolates the individual. Relationships break down due to the consequences of addictive behaviour, such as dishonesty, neglect, or emotional volatility. As addiction worsens, the sense of disconnection intensifies, making it harder for individuals to seek help or reconnect with their communities and loved ones.

Why it happens

Humans are inherently social beings. Our need for connection is fundamental to our wellbeing. When this need goes unmet, it creates a vacuum that can be filled with addictive behaviours such as drinking alcohol, over-eating, excess computer or social media use... etc. Addiction temporarily numbs the pain of disconnection, although it also reinforces feelings of isolation, making recovery more difficult.

What to do

Rebuilding connections is crucial in overcoming addiction. This involves not only reconnecting with family, friends, and society but also fostering a deeper connection with oneself. Engaging in support groups, therapy, and community activities can help restore these vital bonds, providing the social and emotional support necessary for recovery.

3. Addiction and dishonesty

Addiction and dishonesty are deeply intertwined. Dishonesty, both towards oneself and others, is often a hallmark of addictive behaviour. Whether it is hiding substance use, lying about its severity, or denying its impact, dishonesty perpetuates addiction.

How dishonesty maintains addiction

The nature of addiction often leads individuals to conceal their behaviour. This can range from small lies about how much they've consumed to complete denial of having a problem at all. Dishonesty allows addiction to flourish in secrecy, avoiding the scrutiny and intervention that might otherwise interrupt the addictive cycle.

Self-deception is also common. Addicts often tell themselves that they can quit at any time, that they are in control, or that their behaviour isn't harming anyone. These lies act as a shield, protecting the individual from the painful reality of addiction and the need for change.

How it happens

Addiction thrives in environments where truth is obscured. Dishonesty serves as a coping mechanism to avoid the guilt, shame, and fear associated with addiction. Lying to others prevents confrontation, while lying to oneself delays the need for action. However, this dishonesty only deepens the problem, making recovery more difficult.

What to do

Honesty is a cornerstone of recovery. Acknowledging the reality of addiction, both to oneself and others, is the first step towards change. Support groups and therapy provide a safe space for individuals to confront their addiction openly and without judgement. Cultivating honesty helps dismantle the denial that sustains addiction and enables individuals to seek the help they need.

4. Addiction and distraction

In an increasingly fast-paced and overstimulated world, distraction has become both a trigger and a consequence of addiction. Many individuals turn to addictive behaviours or substances to escape the pressures of life, using them as a distraction from deeper emotional issues or uncomfortable realities. (See Chapter 34 on Boredom.)

How distraction contributes to addiction

Addictive substances and behaviours provide an immediate escape from stress, anxiety, and emotional pain. Whether it's scrolling endlessly through social media, binge drinking, or gambling, these behaviours offer temporary relief from life's challenges. Addiction to distraction can quickly spiral, as the need to escape intensifies with each use.

In many cases, addiction serves as a way to avoid confronting deeper issues, such as unresolved trauma, relationship problems, or dissatisfaction with life. Rather than facing these challenges, individuals become trapped in a cycle of distraction, using addiction to numb themselves to their underlying pain.

How it happens

The human brain is wired to seek pleasure and avoid pain. Distraction through addiction offers immediate gratification and relief, even if it is short lived. This cycle of seeking temporary escape is perpetuated by modern society, where quick fixes and instant gratification are readily available.

What to do

Breaking free from addiction to distraction requires mindfulness and self-awareness. Learning to sit with uncomfortable feelings and confront life's challenges head-on is essential. Practices such as meditation, therapy, and journaling can help individuals develop the emotional resilience needed to face difficulties without turning to addictive distractions.

5. Addiction and detachment

Detachment, or emotional numbing, is a common response in addiction. As addiction deepens, individuals often become detached from their emotions, their relationships, and even their sense of self. This detachment not only perpetuates addiction; it also prevents recovery. (See Chapter 27 on Relationships.)

How detachment reinforces addiction

Addiction often leads to emotional numbing as a way to avoid the pain, guilt, or shame associated with the behaviour. As addiction progresses, individuals may become detached from their emotions altogether, using substances or behaviours to suppress their feelings. This detachment creates a barrier between the individual and the world, making it difficult to engage meaningfully in relationships, work, or personal growth.

Detachment from oneself is also common. Addiction can erode self-awareness, making it difficult for individuals to recognise the impact of their behaviour or take responsibility for their actions. This emotional distance further isolates them, perpetuating the cycle of addiction.

How it happens

Detachment serves as a defence mechanism in addiction. Facing the reality of addiction can be overwhelming, and detaching from emotions or relationships offers a temporary reprieve. However, this detachment ultimately deepens the addiction, as the individual becomes increasingly disconnected from the world around them.

What to do

Healing detachment involves reconnecting with emotions and fostering a deeper sense of self-awareness. Therapy, particularly approaches such as cognitive behavioural therapy (CBT) or dialectical behaviour therapy (DBT) (see Chapters 44 and 45), can help individuals re-engage with their emotions and develop healthier coping strategies. Re-establishing emotional connections with loved ones and finding a sense of purpose in life are also key components of recovery.

When to act

As I've said before, the time to act is *now*. Whether you are struggling with addiction yourself or supporting someone on their journey, recognising the interconnected nature of these elements is crucial. Early intervention, honesty, and reconnection - both with oneself and others - are essential for breaking free from the cycle.

> **My personal experience**
>
> What I didn't realise for a long time was how interconnected everything was. My overworking wasn't just affecting one part of my life - it was impacting my health, relationships, and emotional state. The ripple effect was far-reaching. Understanding this interconnected web helped me approach my reset in a more holistic way. I realised that in order to heal, I needed to address not just one area of my life; it was every aspect that had been affected. I could no longer ignore how all these areas were entwined, and that awareness became a crucial part of my reset.

Conclusion

Addiction is not just about substance abuse or compulsive behaviours; it is deeply rooted in a web of disease, disconnection, dishonesty, distraction, and detachment. These elements are not isolated; they feed into each other, creating a cycle that traps individuals in the grip of addiction.

By addressing the root causes of addiction and fostering a holistic approach to recovery, individuals can begin to untangle the web of addiction and move towards healing, wholeness, and freedom.

CHAPTER 7

CROSS-ADDICTION: UNDERSTANDING THE TIES THAT BIND

Addiction is a complex condition, characterised by compulsive engagement in rewarding stimuli, despite adverse consequences. While many people think of addiction as a singular problem - with alcohol, drugs, gambling, food, sex, or even exercise - it is far more complicated. Cross-addiction, also known as addiction transfer, occurs when an individual with one form of addiction switches to another, often unconsciously. This chapter will explore why and how cross-addiction happens, the underlying connections between different addictive behaviours, and what steps can be taken to prevent or manage it.

Understanding what cross-addiction is

Cross-addiction refers to the process where a person recovers from one addiction only to develop a new one. This can involve moving from one substance (e.g. alcohol) to another (e.g. prescription medication), or from substance use to behavioural addictions, such as gambling, shopping, or excessive exercise. It is crucial to understand that cross-addiction is not simply a relapse into the original behaviour; it is rather the emergence of a new compulsive behaviour that offers similar psychological rewards. (See also Chapter 10 on relapse in addiction.)

How it happens

The underlying mechanisms that contribute to addiction - such as brain chemistry, emotional regulation, and coping mechanisms - are often shared across various forms of addiction. Here's how cross-addiction happens:

1. **Shared neurological pathways:** Addiction affects the brain's reward system, particularly the release of dopamine, a neurotransmitter associated with pleasure and motivation. Whether it's alcohol, drugs, or gambling, these addictive behaviours all trigger this reward system, leading to a sense of euphoria. When an individual stops engaging in one addiction, the brain still craves that dopamine release. If the underlying issues that fuelled the original addiction remain unaddressed, it becomes easy to replace one addiction with another.

2. **The role of habit loops:** Addictions are often driven by habit loops, which involve a cue (a trigger for a behaviour), the routine (the behaviour itself), and the reward (the sense of relief or pleasure). When someone removes the original behaviour (e.g. drinking alcohol), the brain is still wired to seek out the reward. Without addressing the trigger and reward dynamics, the individual may adopt a new behaviour (e.g. gambling or shopping) to complete the loop.

3. **Emotional regulation and coping mechanisms:** Many addictions develop as coping strategies for stress, anxiety, depression, trauma, or other emotional pain. When a

person stops using one substance or behaviour to cope, they may feel emotionally vulnerable. If they haven't developed healthier ways to manage their emotions, they are likely to reach for another form of relief, resulting in cross-addiction.

4. **Addictive personality traits:** Some individuals are more predisposed to addiction because of certain personality traits, such as impulsivity, a need for instant gratification, or risk-taking behaviour. These traits don't just disappear after recovering from one addiction. Without proper intervention, these tendencies can manifest in other compulsive behaviours.

Why there is a connection between different addictions

Though various addictions may seem unrelated on the surface – for example, alcohol abuse versus compulsive shopping – they are often deeply connected. The core issue isn't the specific substance or behaviour, it is the individual's inability to regulate their behaviour in relation to stress, reward, and emotional pain.

This inability may arise for one or more of the following reasons:

1. **The brain's wiring:** The brain doesn't differentiate between different addictions; it simply craves the chemical reward of dopamine. Once the brain has been conditioned to seek out and rely on external stimuli for pleasure and relief, it becomes vulnerable to other addictions, regardless of the form.

2. **Psychological need for escape:** Many addictions are rooted in an individual's need to escape from reality. Whether they are avoiding emotional pain, trauma, or daily stressors, the addiction serves as a way to temporarily remove themselves from discomfort. This need for escape can be satisfied by multiple substances or behaviours, meaning the shift from

one addiction to another is often seamless.

3. **Underlying mental health issues:** Co-occurring mental health disorders (such as anxiety, depression, or PTSD) are common among individuals with addiction. These disorders often remain untreated even when someone seeks help for their addiction, leading to cross-addiction. As long as the mental health condition is untreated or unmanaged, the likelihood of seeking relief in a new addiction remains high.

What to do to prevent or address cross-addiction

Managing cross-addiction requires a comprehensive approach that goes beyond simply quitting a substance or behaviour. It involves addressing the root causes of addiction, creating healthy coping mechanisms, and building resilience. Here are some key strategies:

1. **Holistic treatment:** Recovery from addiction should focus not just on stopping the problematic behaviour, but on healing the whole person. This involves treating the underlying psychological, emotional, and physical issues. Cognitive behavioural therapy (CBT), mindfulness-based therapies, and holistic practices such as yoga or meditation can help individuals gain control over their impulses and find balance in their lives.

2. **Focus on emotional and mental health:** Therapy and counselling should address the emotional reasons behind addiction. It's vital to explore issues such as trauma, stress, self-esteem, and relationships, which often fuel addictive behaviours. Learning healthier ways to process emotions reduces the need for addictive substances or activities.

3. **Building healthy coping mechanisms:** Teaching

individuals new ways to cope with stress, anxiety, and emotional pain is a critical part of preventing cross-addiction. This could involve practising relaxation techniques, engaging in physical activity, or developing hobbies that provide a healthy sense of accomplishment and satisfaction.

4. **Support networks:** Having a solid support network is vital for recovery. Whether it's a 12-step programme, counselling group, or trusted friends and family, the encouragement and guidance of others can help keep someone accountable and on track. Support groups specifically for cross-addiction can also be helpful, as they provide insight into the shared experiences of those who have dealt with multiple addictions.

5. **Mindful recovery:** Recovery is not a one-size-fits-all process. It requires ongoing self-awareness, particularly in recognising the warning signs of cross-addiction. Mindfulness practices, such as meditation or journaling, can help individuals identify triggers and behaviours before they escalate into a new addiction.

When to act

Recognising cross-addiction is crucial in preventing its progression. It's important to be vigilant for signs such as:

- Shifting focus from one addiction to another (e.g. stopping substance abuse and then developing compulsive gambling habits).
- Using new behaviours or substances to cope with stress, boredom, or emotional pain.
- Feeling the same sense of loss of control over the new behaviour or substance as with the original addiction.

If these signs emerge, it's essential to seek help immediately. Taking early action can prevent a new addiction from becoming entrenched and more difficult to treat. Revisiting treatment programmes, increasing therapy sessions, or joining support groups focused on addiction management, can be highly beneficial.

Conclusion

Cross-addiction highlights the fact that addiction is not simply about the substance or behaviour; it is about deeper psychological, emotional, and neurological issues. Preventing or managing cross-addiction requires addressing these root causes, creating healthier coping mechanisms, and fostering self-awareness. By recognising the connections between different addictions and understanding how they develop, individuals can build a more sustainable recovery, one that is free from the bonds of addiction transfer.

CHAPTER 8

HIGH-FUNCTIONING ADDICTION: THE MASK BEHIND THE SUCCESS

Addiction is commonly visualised as catastrophic - unemployment, estrangement from family, criminal behaviour, or health deterioration. These images, though accurate in some cases, fail to reflect the quieter, more insidious form of addiction that thrives behind competence, routine, and professional success: high-functioning addiction. This chapter explores the nature of high-functioning addiction, how it takes root, why it persists unnoticed, and the steps necessary to recognise and address it.

What high-functioning addiction is

High-functioning addiction describes individuals who maintain the appearance of stability while living with a dependency on substances or behaviours. They meet deadlines, lead meetings, raise children, and fulfil social obligations. From the outside, their lives appear orderly, even aspirational. Behind closed doors, however, they are reliant on a substance (such as alcohol, stimulants, or prescription medication) or a behaviour (such as gambling, sex, or compulsive work) to regulate their emotional state, maintain performance, or escape discomfort.

This form of addiction is particularly difficult to detect, both by others and by the individual themselves. Functioning becomes a mask - an armour that hides internal distress, slowly eroding wellbeing from within.

How it happens

High-functioning addiction doesn't emerge out of nowhere. It is usually the result of a gradual shift - one drink to unwind becomes two, a bit of pressure relief becomes a nightly ritual, and suddenly, functioning without the behaviour feels impossible. Understanding the conditions that foster this form of addiction is key to identifying it early. From high-pressure jobs and cultural norms to personal traits and coping mechanisms, several interlocking factors can quietly lead someone into dependence while life on the surface appears untouched.

1. **Social and professional demands:** Many careers demand perfection, long hours, and constant availability. High-functioning addicts often operate in environments that reward intensity - whether that's a law firm, hospital, financial institution, or creative industry. The pace and pressure are relentless, and substances may begin as tools for endurance: a glass of wine to unwind, a pill to stay alert, or a stimulant to boost confidence. Eventually, these tools become necessary just to maintain the standard. What started as a choice becomes a dependency. And in some industries, substance use is part of the culture. Colleagues gather at the pub after work, late-night shifts are fuelled by caffeine and energy drinks, and stress is normalised rather than treated.

2. **Cultural norms and acceptance:** In UK society, alcohol in particular holds a strong cultural presence. Celebrations,

commiserations, networking events, and even charity fundraisers often involve drinking. This makes excessive use easy to hide, especially if everyone else is doing the same. The phrase 'everyone's a bit stressed' can be used to dismiss real struggles. Similarly, someone who drinks a bottle of wine each night may not be questioned if they continue to perform well during the day.

3. **Illusion of control:** Functioning addicts are often the last to recognise their problem. They point to their achievements, responsibilities, or productivity as evidence that everything is under control. This belief not only delays self-awareness; it can also be reinforced by others who admire or depend on that person.

The illusion of control is dangerous. While the person may still be functioning outwardly, the cost is growing - physically, emotionally, and psychologically.

Why there is a connection between high achievement and addiction

It may seem paradoxical that individuals who are successful, driven, and outwardly in control are vulnerable to addiction, yet the very traits that lead to high performance - perfectionism, self-discipline, ambition - can also become risk factors. When external achievement masks internal stress or emotional neglect, substances or behaviours may be used to fill the gap. In this section, we explore why high achievers often walk a fine line between excellence and self-destruction, and how the overlap between capability and vulnerability can leave addiction hidden in plain sight.

There is a striking overlap between personality traits associated with high achievement and those that increase vulnerability to addiction.

1. **Perfectionism and pressure:** Perfectionism drives people to set impossibly high standards for themselves. When these standards are not met - or even when they are - there is little space for self-compassion. Substances become a way to soothe the chronic tension.

2. **The self-reliance shield:** Self-reliance and fear of vulnerability often mean individuals do not seek help or share struggles. They internalise pressure, fearing that honesty about their challenges will lead to judgement or weakness.

3. **Imposter syndrome's grip:** Imposter syndrome, common among professionals, fuels insecurity. The feeling of not being 'good enough' despite evidence to the contrary can lead to anxiety, burnout, and emotional depletion. Many turn to substances to fill that emotional void or to maintain the illusion of competence.

4. **Driven by impulse:** Reward-seeking and impulsivity - traits that sometimes drive entrepreneurs and creatives - can also make addictive behaviours more appealing and harder to resist.

The same qualities that drive excellence can turn destructive without balance, boundaries, and healthy coping strategies.

Why delay is risky

Many high-functioning addicts delay seeking help because their lives still appear manageable. They may not have experienced public failure or severe consequences, and so the urgency to change doesn't feel immediate. This delay is one of the greatest dangers.

Addiction is progressive – it doesn't stand still. What seems under control today can spiral tomorrow. In this section, we explore why waiting to address high-functioning addiction allows the condition to deepen and why early action, even in the absence of crisis, can make recovery more effective and less painful.

1. **The physical:** Physically, the body begins to suffer, even when outward signs are subtle at first. Alcohol and other substances place strain on key organs, especially the liver and heart. Sleep becomes fragmented or non-restorative, energy levels drop, and mental clarity diminishes. Over time, the body adapts to the presence of the substance, leading to increased tolerance and the need for more to achieve the same effect. These changes are often gradual, making them easy to overlook until the physical toll becomes undeniable.

2. **The psychological:** Psychologically, addiction alters the way the mind processes reality. It fosters denial, rationalisation, and minimisation of risk. Emotional numbness or avoidance becomes a default setting, making it harder to connect authentically with others. Even in the absence of overt conflict, relationships begin to suffer due to growing withdrawal, irritability, or emotional unavailability. The person may still be physically present, yet psychologically distant, lost in thought, anxiety, or preoccupation with their next use.

3. **The professional:** Professionally, the impact of addiction eventually becomes harder to conceal. The individual may begin missing small details, making uncharacteristic mistakes, or struggling with punctuality. Their emotional responses may shift – becoming more reactive, short-tempered, or distant under pressure. As stress accumulates and

cognitive functioning declines, the polished exterior begins to crack. What once felt effortless becomes a performance that requires increasing effort to maintain.

High-functioning addiction often collapses slowly, then suddenly. The breakdown of health, relationships, or work performance can happen with little warning, shocking both the individual and those around them.

Early intervention significantly improves outcomes. It prevents crises and allows for recovery to begin from a place of strength rather than collapse.

Recognising the signs

High-functioning addiction can be incredibly difficult to detect because it often coexists with success, charm, and apparent normality. However, there are always signs, some subtle, others more pronounced, that indicate something is out of balance. Recognising these early can mean the difference between prolonged suffering and timely support. Whether you're concerned about yourself or someone else, this section outlines the behavioural and emotional patterns that suggest functioning is starting to come at too great a cost.

High-functioning addiction doesn't always resemble the stereotypical images we see in the media or academic literature. Rather than dramatic collapse, it often develops gradually. More often, it's hidden beneath routines and rationalisations, social norms, and outward success. The signs develop slowly and subtly, easy to overlook, even by the person experiencing them:

1. **Routine substance use to regulate emotions:** Using alcohol, stimulants, or sedatives to manage energy, mood, or

stress becomes a daily habit. Over time, reliance grows, not for pleasure, but to feel 'normal' or stable.

2. **Preoccupied thoughts:** Even when not using, there's frequent mental space given to planning the next opportunity, managing logistics, or craving relief. It gradually shapes focus and daily decisions.

3. **Increased secrecy:** Usage becomes something to conceal. Bottles may be hidden, quantities downplayed, or behaviours explained away. Defensiveness often replaces openness with others.

4. **Performance anxiety:** A creeping fear of not being able to cope without the substance or behaviour emerges. Work, social life, or even rest feels harder without the usual coping aid.

5. **Loss of pleasure in normal activities:** Things that were once enjoyable feel flat. Increasingly, the only activity that brings relief or stimulation is the addictive one, even if it no longer feels especially good.

6. **Emotional volatility:** Mood swings, anxiety, or irritability appear more often, with no obvious cause. This can be linked to withdrawal, stress, or the effort of holding everything together.

7. **Rationalisation:** Thoughts like 'I deserve this' or 'It's under control' help to maintain the habit. Because life still appears functional, the problem is easier to dismiss or deny.

8. **Reward framing:** The behaviour is viewed as a reward for hard work or stress. This reinforces its place in daily life and normalises patterns that might otherwise raise concern.

Family, friends, and colleagues may notice these shifts long before the person does. Consistency over time, not isolated events, paints the clearest picture.

When to seek help

Facing high-functioning addiction can feel overwhelming, especially when so much of life appears intact. Yet the decision to seek help or offer support doesn't require things to fall apart first. In fact, the earlier the intervention, the more intact a person's life remains through the recovery process. This section offers practical guidance for individuals who suspect they may be struggling, as well as for those concerned about someone close to them. Timing matters, and knowing what to do, and when, can make all the difference.

If you are struggling:

1. **Acknowledge the impact your use is having:** Notice how your use is affecting you, even if it hasn't yet caused obvious damage. You don't need to hit 'rock bottom' for your experience to be valid. Subtle shifts, strained relationships, rising anxiety, poor sleep, or numbness, are worth noticing. Being honest with yourself is the first step toward change.
2. **Track your patterns:** Track what, when, and why you use. Patterns reveal function. Understanding your behaviour helps reduce shame and build insight. Paying attention to what precedes use can reveal stressors, triggers, and unmet needs calling for healthier responses.
3. **Speak to someone:** Reach out to someone, not necessarily with a full confession, but with complete honesty. A therapist, GP, or trusted friend can provide perspective and support. You don't need all the answers before seeking help. Saying 'I'm struggling more than I let on' can open a door.

Choose someone who can listen without judgement.

4. **Avoid waiting for a disaster:** Recovery does not require collapse; it begins with awareness and willingness. You're allowed to act before things fall apart. Early action often leads to better outcomes. Recovery is a move toward something better, not a consequence of failure.

If you are concerned about someone else:

1. **Choose your moment carefully:** Speak with calm and compassion, not confrontation. Timing and tone matter. A quiet, low-stress moment invites openness. Confrontation can create resistance, while steady presence builds trust.
2. **Focus on behaviours, not labels:** 'You've seemed more anxious lately,' rather than 'You're drinking too much.' Observations invite reflection, whereas labels can feel like attacks. Avoid naming or diagnosing. Share what you've noticed and give the person room to respond.
3. **Offer support, not solutions:** Suggest options, listen openly, and create a safe space for the person to reflect. You're not there to prescribe. Simple words - such as, 'You're not alone' or 'There's help if you want it,' can be powerful. Let the person move at their own pace.
4. **Be consistent:** Denial is common. Your calm concern may plant a seed that grows later. They may not respond right away. They may reject your concern. Stay calm and caring. Your quiet presence might become the support they turn to when they're ready.

The ideal moment for intervention is early, before the addiction undermines health, relationships, or career. That said, the right moment is also whenever awareness breaks through. Whether that comes after a mistake, an illness, or a moment of reflection, the opportunity for recovery is always present.

Intervening early reduces shame, preserves self-esteem, and increases the chance of sustained recovery.

Treatment options

Recovery from high-functioning addiction is not one-size-fits-all. The demands of daily life, career responsibilities, and personal privacy mean that many individuals require tailored treatment approaches that fit their circumstances. Fortunately, a range of effective and flexible options are available. This section outlines the various forms of treatment, from therapy and outpatient programmes to specialist rehabilitation centres and integrated care, highlighting that meaningful recovery is not only possible; it is also adaptable to individual needs.

1. **Outpatient counselling and therapy:** Outpatient therapy allows individuals to access support while continuing with daily life. Sessions can be scheduled flexibly, with approaches like CBT (see Chapter 44), DBT (see Chapter 39), or trauma-informed therapy (see Chapter 13) used to explore the roots of addiction and build healthier coping strategies.

2. **Executive or professional rehab programmes:** These specialised programmes are designed for those in high-pressure roles. They offer confidential, tailored treatment in settings that respect privacy, often with flexibility to maintain some work commitments during recovery. Often, these programmes are set in beautiful surroundings with a luxurious feel to them.

3. **Group therapy and peer support:** Structured peer groups, such as SMART Recovery or executive-focused 12-step meetings, create space for connection and accountability. Sharing experiences with others in similar situations helps

to reduce isolation and to build trust.

4. **Integrated and holistic care:** Addiction often overlaps with anxiety, depression, trauma, or burnout. A well-rounded approach treats both the substance use and the underlying issues, supporting long-term healing through medical, psychological, and emotional care.

Long-term support is essential. Recovery is a process, not a single event, and requires sustained care, reflection, and connection.

Conclusion

The term 'high-functioning' can be deeply misleading. It implies strength, competence, and success, yet beneath the surface it often conceals emotional distress and growing dependence. Functioning, in this context, is not the same as flourishing - it is a performance that drains emotional, physical, and psychological reserves. Those who appear in control may, in reality, be operating from a place of fear, pain, or deep exhaustion. High-functioning addiction is not sustainable. Over time, the effort to maintain the façade becomes increasingly costly, chipping away at a person's wellbeing and sense of self.

Recovery, however, is possible at any stage. It does not require collapse or crisis to begin - only the courage to recognise that surviving is not the same as thriving. The process is not about losing identity; it is about reclaiming it. The energy once spent on managing appearances can be redirected toward healing, authenticity, and lasting wellbeing. True freedom lies not in hiding pain, but in facing it with honesty - supported by those who see beyond the performance and into the person beneath. In that space, the opportunity for genuine connection, renewal, and sustainable success is finally allowed to take root.

CHAPTER 9

ADDICTION FOR LIFE: UNDERSTANDING LIFELONG CONNECTIONS

Addiction is often portrayed as a battle that can be won with the right tools and enough perseverance. However, for many, addiction is not a battle that ever fully ends; it is a condition that requires constant vigilance and long-term management. When we speak of addiction for life, we are addressing a multifaceted relationship between an individual and the object of their addiction - be it substances, behaviours, or even emotional dependencies - that can persist indefinitely, despite periods of recovery. In this chapter, we will explore how lifelong addiction forms, why it happens, the mechanisms that strengthen the connection, and what strategies can be employed to manage it effectively.

How addiction becomes a lifelong struggle

Addiction can be likened to a chronic illness such as diabetes or heart disease. Like these conditions, addiction has both genetic and environmental factors, as well as physical, psychological, and social components. The process of becoming addicted starts with the interaction between a person's brain chemistry and an addictive substance or behaviour. Over time, repeated exposure to a substance or behaviour alters brain function, particularly in the reward system.

At its core, addiction hijacks the brain's reward system, which is responsible for the regulation of pleasure and motivation. Normally, this system encourages behaviours necessary for survival, such as eating and social bonding. However, substances like alcohol, drugs, and even activities like gambling or social media use, can produce feelings of pleasure so intense that the brain begins to prioritise these artificial sources of reward above all else.

Even after detoxification and extended periods of sobriety, these changes in brain chemistry can persist, making relapse a real risk. Just as someone with diabetes cannot ignore their condition, someone with a history of addiction often faces the possibility of relapse, even years after achieving recovery. This is what makes addiction a lifelong challenge – it is not just a behavioural issue; it is a rewiring of the brain.

Why lifelong addiction happens

Addiction for life is not merely the result of individual choices; it arises from a combination of genetic, psychological, and environmental factors. In this section, we explore the underlying reasons why addiction can last a lifetime, from inherited predispositions to deep-rooted psychological vulnerabilities.

There are a number of factors that contribute to addiction becoming a lifelong struggle:

1. **Genetic predisposition:** Research suggests that genetics play a significant role in the development of addiction. If addiction runs in a family, it is more likely that members of

future generations will also experience it. Some people are biologically wired to become addicted more easily than others. They may have lower levels of dopamine, the chemical responsible for pleasure and reward, or they may metabolise substances differently. This predisposition doesn't guarantee addiction although it increases susceptibility.

2. **Psychological vulnerabilities:** Addiction often serves as a coping mechanism for underlying psychological conditions such as anxiety, depression, trauma, or stress. These conditions can be long-term, requiring continual management and care. For many, addiction becomes a way to numb painful emotions or escape unresolved trauma. Even after substance use stops, the underlying psychological issues may persist, making lifelong management essential.

3. **Environmental influences:** Environmental factors, such as growing up in a household where substance abuse is normalised or experiencing chronic stress, can play a pivotal role in the development of lifelong addiction. Social and cultural influences, including peer pressure and media representation, also reinforce addictive behaviours. In some cases, people become stuck in cycles of addiction because their environments never change, limiting their ability to break free from unhealthy patterns.

4. **Neuroplasticity and memory:** The brain's ability to adapt and change (neuroplasticity) means that addictive behaviours become deeply ingrained over time. When a person engages in an addictive behaviour repeatedly, neural pathways strengthen, making it easier to fall back into that behaviour in the future. Even after abstaining for years, certain triggers - such as stress, emotional distress, or exposure to the substance - can reawaken these pathways. This is

why someone can relapse after decades of sobriety.

What makes the connection so strong

The power of addiction lies in its ability to create strong, persistent connections in the brain, making it difficult to sever the ties between a person and their addictive substance or behaviour. Here, we examine the mechanisms that make addiction so deeply ingrained, including conditioned responses, reward cycles, and tolerance.

Several factors contribute to the deep and persistent connection between an individual and their addiction:

1. **Conditioned response:** As someone becomes addicted, their brain learns to associate certain environments, people, or situations with the substance or behaviour. This conditioning creates powerful associations that can be difficult to break. A pub might trigger a craving for alcohol, or stress at work might lead someone to reach for a cigarette. These connections persist long after physical dependence has been overcome.

2. **The cycle of reward and punishment:** Addiction often follows a cycle of reward and punishment. Initially, engaging in the addictive behaviour brings pleasure and relief, but over time, continued use leads to negative consequences, such as health issues, relationship problems, or financial difficulties. Despite these negative outcomes, the brain continues to seek the reward because it has become dependent on the substance or behaviour for pleasure and relief.

3. **Escalation and tolerance:** Over time, the body becomes tolerant to the effects of a substance or behaviour, requiring more of it to achieve the same level of pleasure or relief. This

leads to a dangerous cycle where the individual increases their consumption, further strengthening the addiction. This tolerance creates a sense of entrapment, where the individual feels compelled to continue using despite the consequences.

What to do

Managing lifelong addiction requires a multifaceted approach. While complete recovery is possible, it often involves continuous maintenance and vigilance. Here are some key strategies for managing lifelong addiction:

1. **Acknowledge the chronic nature of addiction:** The first step is to accept that addiction is a chronic condition, much like hypertension or asthma. It requires long-term care and management rather than a one-time solution. Understanding this can reduce feelings of guilt or failure if a relapse occurs.

2. **Develop a support network:** Support from others is crucial in managing lifelong addiction. This can include family, friends, therapists, support groups, or recovery communities. Having people who understand your struggles and offer encouragement is often the key to maintaining long-term recovery.

3. **Therapeutic interventions:** Various forms of therapy, such as cognitive behavioural therapy (CBT), mindfulness-based relapse prevention, or trauma-informed therapy, can be beneficial for addressing the underlying causes of addiction. Therapy helps individuals develop coping mechanisms and strategies for dealing with triggers and stressors that may lead to relapse.

4. **Adopt a holistic approach:** Lifelong addiction management often requires a holistic approach that addresses not only the physical aspects of addiction, but also the emotional, social, and spiritual components. Practices such as meditation, mindfulness, yoga, and physical exercise can help balance the body and mind.

5. **Set realistic goals:** Setting realistic goals, such as reducing harm rather than aiming for total abstinence, may be necessary for some people. While abstinence is the ideal outcome, harm reduction strategies (such as limiting substance use or switching to less harmful alternatives) can help reduce the negative impacts of addiction.

When to act

The time to act is as soon as addiction is recognised, whether it is in yourself or a loved one. Early intervention often leads to better outcomes. However, it is never too late to seek help. Recovery can begin at any stage, and even after decades of addiction, change is possible.

If you notice that cravings are becoming more frequent, or that you are increasingly preoccupied with thoughts of substance use or addictive behaviour, these are signs that immediate action is needed. Seeking professional help, whether through a therapist, addiction specialist, or support group, is crucial.

My personal experience

For me, going through recovery or a personal reset leaves a lasting imprint. The insights you gain – the unravelling of old patterns - don't simply disappear. You don't forget the thoughts or emotions that once surfaced; instead, you become more attuned to them. You are more aware of how you feel, and often, why you feel that way. If that awareness isn't yet clear, or has started to wane, it can be a sign that deeper self-reflection and understanding is still needed. I believe this awareness remains with you, for as long as you choose to live in alignment with your values and the person you've become.

Conclusion

Addiction for life is a reality for many individuals. Though it is challenging, it is not insurmountable. With the right tools, support, and a commitment to long-term management, it is possible to live a fulfilling life while navigating the complexities of addiction. While the path may not always be linear, and relapses may occur, each step towards recovery strengthens resilience. Ultimately, lifelong addiction management is about accepting the condition, understanding its mechanisms, and building a strategy that allows for continual growth, healing, and hope.

CHAPTER 10

UNDERSTANDING RELAPSE IN ADDICTION

Relapse is often viewed as a setback, a step backwards on the road to recovery. However, in the realm of addiction, relapse is not merely a failure – it's often part of the journey. Recovery is not a linear process. Understanding relapse, why it happens, and how to respond to it, is a vital aspect of overcoming addiction. In this chapter, we delve into what makes relapse such a common experience in addiction, why it happens, and how to navigate through it constructively.

What relapse is

Relapse is typically defined as the return to substance use after a period of abstinence. However, it can also refer to returning to any addictive behaviour, whether related to substances, gambling, or other compulsive actions. It's important to understand that relapse is not a single even; it is a process that happens over time. This process is often broken down into three stages:

1. **Emotional relapse:** At this stage, the individual may not be consciously thinking about using; however, they begin to experience emotions and behaviours that make them vulnerable to relapse. Anxiety, irritability, isolation, or

neglecting self-care may be early warning signs. The individual may start distancing themselves from support systems or routines that kept them on the path of recovery.

2. **Mental relapse:** Here, the battle between recovery and the desire to use again begins. Thoughts about using, romanticising past behaviour, or justifying why one 'deserves' to indulge may start creeping in. At this point, the individual might be wrestling with cravings, fantasising about using, or even planning a relapse while trying to maintain control.

3. **Physical relapse:** This is the stage where the individual returns to substance use or the addictive behaviour. It can be a one-time occurrence, or it can escalate into full-blown dependence again.

Understanding relapse as a process allows us to intervene earlier – ideally before it reaches the physical stage.

Why relapse happens

Relapse occurs for a variety of reasons, and it is often triggered by a combination of emotional, psychological, and environmental factors. The following are some common reasons people relapse:

1. **Stress:** Life stressors are a major contributor to relapse. Problems at work, relationship issues, financial strain, or unresolved trauma can trigger an overwhelming desire to escape through old habits of substance use or other addictive behaviours.

2. **Emotional triggers:** Emotions such as anger, loneliness, fear, or sadness can be powerful triggers. These emotions may lead individuals to seek comfort or numbness, especially if they haven't developed healthier coping mechanisms. High

levels of stress and emotion may seem unmanageable, making the appeal of the addictive behaviour stronger.

3. **Overconfidence:** Ironically, success in recovery can sometimes be a risk factor for relapse. After a period of abstinence, people may feel overly confident in their ability to manage their addiction, believing they can re-engage with the substance or behaviour without falling into old patterns. This leads to risky situations where temptations are underestimated.

4. **Social pressure:** Even with the best intentions, social situations can lead to relapse. Being in environments where the substance or behaviour is present, or where peers engage in addictive behaviours, can reignite cravings and make it difficult to resist.

5. **Neglecting self-care:** Recovery requires maintaining a balanced life that includes physical, emotional, and mental wellbeing. When individuals stop engaging in self-care – such as exercising, eating well, attending support groups, or practising mindfulness – they become vulnerable to relapse.

6. **Isolation:** Addiction thrives in isolation, and relapse is more likely when individuals disconnect from their support networks. Without the accountability or encouragement from others, the internal struggle to remain abstinent becomes more challenging.

The connection between relapse and recovery

Relapse is often perceived as a failure, but it's important to reframe this perception. In reality, many people relapse during their recovery – it's part of the learning curve. The journey of recovery involves understanding one's triggers, building resilience, and developing the tools needed to cope with life without the crutch of addiction. Each relapse, while painful, can be an opportunity to reflect on what led to the return of the behaviour and what strategies can be improved going forward.

Recovery is rarely a straight line. The cycles of progress, relapse, and recommitment are part of understanding what long-term sobriety looks like. Many people who successfully overcome addiction experience one or more relapses before they find lasting success. It is not an indication that the person will never recover; it is rather that more insight and tools are required to sustain change.

What to do

If a relapse occurs, the most important thing is to address it swiftly and with compassion. Feelings of shame, guilt, or failure can prevent people from seeking help; however, these emotions only perpetuate the cycle. Here's what to do if a relapse happens:

1. **Acknowledge it:** The first step is to recognise and acknowledge the relapse. Denial will only prolong the process of getting back on track. It's crucial to be honest with oneself and with any support network about what happened.

2. **Avoid self-blame:** Relapse is not a moral failing. Beating oneself up over the relapse only compounds negative emotions, increasing the likelihood of further use. Instead, approach the situation with self-compassion. Everyone makes mistakes, and recovery is about learning and growing from them.

3. **Reach out for support:** Connection is key. Speak to a sponsor, therapist, or trusted friend. If attending a support

group, such as Alcoholics Anonymous (AA) or Narcotics Anonymous (NA), consider increasing the frequency of meetings. Surrounding oneself with supportive people can make a tremendous difference in avoiding further use and regaining stability.

4. **Identify the triggers:** Look back at the events, thoughts, or emotions that led up to the relapse. What were the circumstances? Was there a build-up of stress or were you in certain environments that made it difficult to resist? Understanding the triggers helps to develop a plan to manage them in the future.

5. **Revisit the recovery plan:** A relapse signals that something in the recovery strategy may need to be adjusted. This could mean updating coping strategies, attending therapy more regularly, or seeking out additional treatment. It's a good opportunity to refine one's approach to ensure more robust support against future challenges.

6. **Forgive yourself and move forward:** The quicker one accepts the relapse and takes action, the easier it will be to move forward. Holding onto guilt or regret only fuels more addictive behaviours. It's crucial to forgive oneself, recommit to recovery, and recognise the progress that's already been made.

When to seek professional help

In some cases, especially when the relapse is prolonged or severe, it may be necessary to seek professional help. This could involve returning to a rehabilitation programme or engaging in more intensive therapy. If the relapse feels overwhelming or the individual feels stuck in the cycle of use, professional support can provide the tools needed to break the cycle.

It's also important to note that some relapses can be dangerous, particularly when dealing with substances that have significant physiological effects. After a period of abstinence, the body's tolerance decreases, and returning to previous levels of substance use can result in overdose or other serious health issues. Immediate help is critical in such scenarios.

Conclusion

Relapse is not the end of the recovery journey - it is often a part of it. Understanding why relapse happens and how to respond to it can transform what might feel like a failure into an opportunity for growth and renewed commitment. Recovery is about resilience, not perfection, and every step forward, even after a setback, brings one closer to lasting freedom from addiction.

By approaching relapse with understanding, self-compassion, and practical strategies, individuals can emerge stronger and more equipped to continue their journey towards sobriety. Each experience, even those that feel like a step backwards, offers valuable insights into the nature of addiction and the strength required to overcome it.

PART II

THE CONNECTION TO ADDICTION

Addiction is a symptom of an underlying issue. The addiction is the problem, but it's not the root of the problem

Gabor Maté, *In the Realm of Hungry Ghosts: Close Encounters with Addiction* (2008)

PART II(A)

THE CONNECTION TO ADDICTION: HEALTH AND WELLBEING

The greatest wealth is health.

Virgil , Ancient Roman poet, died 21 September 19 BCE

CHAPTER 11

THE CONNECTION BETWEEN ADDICTION AND PHYSICAL HEALTH

Addiction, whether to substances or behaviours, is a multifaceted issue that profoundly affects not only mental health; it can also affect physical wellbeing, an issue introduced in Chapter 6. The connection between addiction and physical health is undeniable, and understanding how, why, and when this connection occurs is vital in addressing the problem, as we saw. This chapter explores in detail the mechanisms that link addiction to physical health issues, the effects of addiction on the body, and strategies for mitigating its impact.

The connection between physical health and addiction

The connection between addiction and physical health is profound, as addiction affects nearly every system in the body. Substances like alcohol, drugs, and tobacco, as well as addictive behaviours, can directly damage vital organs, disrupt the cardiovascular, respiratory, and digestive systems, and weaken the immune response. For instance, prolonged alcohol use can lead to liver disease, while smoking increases the risk of lung and many other cancers and heart disease. Additionally, the lifestyle associated with addiction - poor nutrition, lack of exercise, and neglect of medical care - exacerbates physical health problems. Understanding this connection is essential for addressing addiction holistically, focusing on both recovery and the restoration of physical wellbeing.

Understanding the link between addiction and physical health

At its core, addiction is a chronic brain disorder characterised by compulsive engagement in rewarding stimuli despite adverse consequences. While much attention is often focused on the psychological and social effects of addiction, its toll on physical health is significant and should not be underestimated.

There are two primary pathways through which addiction harms physical health:

1. **Direct physiological impact:** Substances like drugs, alcohol, or even excessive food intake can directly damage organs, disrupt bodily systems, and lead to chronic health conditions.

2. **Indirect consequences:** Addiction often results in poor lifestyle choices, such as neglecting hygiene, ignoring medical care, lack of nutrition, and increased risk of accidents or injuries, all of which can further damage physical health.

Whether the addiction is to nicotine, alcohol, opioids, or behaviours like gambling or binge-eating, there are physical ramifications that can vary in severity depending on the type and duration of the addiction.

Chapter 11

How addiction impacts physical health

Addiction affects the body in many ways, depending on the substance or behaviour. Common effects include damage to organs, weakened immunity, and long-term health issues, emphasising the need for early intervention. However, there are several common threads that run through most addictions:

1. **Neurological effects:** Addiction primarily affects the brain's reward system, particularly involving neurotransmitters like dopamine. (Others incluce oxytocin, serotonin, adrenaline, noradrenaline, vasopressin and the glucocorticoids.) While dopamine plays a key role in pleasure and motivation, addictive substances overstimulate this system, leading to tolerance and dependence. Over time, the brain requires more of the substance to achieve the same effect, resulting in compulsive use. This neurological alteration impacts not just mental health but physical wellbeing, with withdrawal symptoms, cravings, and reduced cognitive function also affecting bodily functions.

2. **Cardiovascular system:** Many addictive substances, particularly stimulants like cocaine and amphetamines, can have a profound impact on the cardiovascular system. They increase heart rate, raise blood pressure, and constrict blood vessels, increasing the risk of heart attacks, strokes, and other cardiovascular conditions. Even alcohol, often regarded as less harmful, can cause high blood pressure, arrhythmias, and cardiomyopathy when consumed in excess.

3. **Respiratory system:** Tobacco addiction is closely linked to numerous respiratory issues, from chronic obstructive pulmonary disease (COPD) to lung cancer. Even non-inhalable substances like opioids can suppress the respiratory system,

leading to conditions such as hypoxia and, in severe cases, respiratory arrest.

4. **Digestive and hepatic systems:** The liver, being responsible for metabolising most drugs and alcohol, is particularly vulnerable to addiction. Chronic alcohol use is a well known cause of liver diseases, including fatty liver, hepatitis, and cirrhosis. Opioid addiction, meanwhile, can cause severe constipation, bowel dysfunction, and malnutrition, impacting digestive health.

5. **Immune system:** Addiction weakens the immune system, making individuals more susceptible to infections and diseases. Alcohol and drugs can suppress immune responses, making it difficult for the body to fight off common illnesses like colds and flu, as well as more serious conditions such as pneumonia and tuberculosis.

6. **Musculoskeletal system:** Chronic use of addictive substances can lead to musculoskeletal problems such as weakened bones, joint pain, and muscle atrophy. For example, long-term alcohol abuse can interfere with calcium absorption, leading to osteoporosis, while drug abuse can cause muscle breakdown (rhabdomyolysis), leading to kidney damage.

7. **Hormonal imbalances:** Substances like alcohol and drugs can disrupt the endocrine system, leading to hormonal imbalances that affect everything from metabolism to reproductive health. This can result in irregular periods in women, reduced testosterone levels in men, and increased risk of infertility.

8. **Cancer risk:** Addiction to certain substances increases the risk of developing cancer. For instance, smoking is one of

the leading causes of lung, throat, and bladder cancers. Alcohol abuse is linked to cancers of the liver, oesophagus, breast, and colon.

How addiction leads to physical health problems

The physical deterioration seen in addiction is often due to the toxic effects of the substances themselves. Most addictive substances are foreign to the body and are treated as toxins. The liver and kidneys are responsible for detoxifying these substances; however, when the intake becomes excessive, the body's ability to process them is overwhelmed, leading to cell damage and disease.

Beyond this, addictive behaviours often lead to neglect of self-care. Individuals may forgo meals, hygiene, exercise, and sleep, which further weakens the body. The constant strain of withdrawal and relapse cycles places additional stress on the body's systems, accelerating wear and tear.

When physical health problems arise

Physical health problems related to addiction can begin almost immediately in some cases. For instance, opioid overdoses can cause instant respiratory failure, while a single instance of binge drinking can lead to alcohol poisoning.

However, in many cases, the physical effects of addiction develop gradually. Chronic health conditions such as liver disease, heart disease, and cancer may take years of substance abuse to manifest, though the body is often suffering from subtle yet cumulative damage in the interim.

The timing of these health problems also depends on factors such as the individual's genetics, the type and amount of substance used, and the duration of addiction. For example, some people may develop lung cancer after a decade of smoking, while others may be affected much later or not at all, though they still face other health risks like COPD.

What to do to mitigate the physical health impact of addiction

The good news is that, with the right interventions, the body can often recover from many of the physical effects of addiction. While the process may be challenging, it is possible to reverse or manage some of the damage. Mitigating these effects requires a comprehensive, multi-faceted approach, involving medical treatment, lifestyle changes, and ongoing support to restore both physical and mental health.

1. **Medical detoxification and treatment:** Detox is the first step to ridding the body of harmful substances, although it must be done under medical supervision, particularly for substances like alcohol and benzodiazepines, where withdrawal can be life-threatening. Following detox, medications may be prescribed to help manage cravings and reduce the likelihood of relapse. For example, methadone or buprenorphine may be used for opioid addiction, while nicotine patches can help smokers quit.

2. **Healthy lifestyle choices:** Restoring physical health also involves adopting healthier habits, such as improving nutrition, exercising regularly, and getting adequate sleep. Proper diet and exercise can help repair damage to the cardiovascular system, reduce inflammation, and support immune function.

3. **Regular medical check-ups:** Addicted individuals should

seek regular medical care to monitor and address any developing health issues. Early detection of conditions like liver disease, high blood pressure, or cancer can significantly improve outcomes.

4. **Mental health support:** Because mental and physical health are interconnected, addressing mental health issues is crucial. Many people struggling with addiction also suffer from anxiety, depression, and/or trauma, which can exacerbate physical health problems. Therapy, support groups, and sometimes psychiatric medication can be essential parts of recovery.

5. **Social support and rehabilitation programmes:** Support from family, friends, and addiction recovery programmes can provide the necessary encouragement to stick with treatment and maintain healthy behaviours. Rehabilitation centres can offer holistic care, addressing both physical and mental aspects of addiction.

When to seek help

Recognising when addiction is taking a significant toll on your physical health is crucial for preventing further harm. If you or someone you know is experiencing any of the following physical health signs, it is important to seek professional assistance to address the effects of addiction on the body.

1. **Physical health deterioration:** Symptoms such as rapid weight loss or gain, constant fatigue, difficulty breathing, or pain in the chest or abdomen may indicate that addiction is severely affecting your vital organs, such as your heart, lungs, or liver.

2. **Health complications from chronic substance use:** Frequent infections, irregular heartbeats, digestive issues, or persistent coughing could suggest that substance use is leading to chronic conditions like respiratory issues, heart disease, or liver damage. Immediate medical attention is necessary to address these complications.

3. **Physical withdrawal symptoms:** Physical signs such as tremors, sweating, nausea, or severe cravings when attempting to stop using a substance often indicate physical dependence. These symptoms signal the need for medically supervised detox to prevent further health risks.

4. **Difficulty in managing physical wellbeing:** Neglecting basic self-care, such as eating, drinking, or sleeping properly due to addiction, can lead to malnutrition, dehydration, and weakened immune function. Seeking help is vital to restoring your physical health.

5. **Signs of organ damage:** Symptoms like jaundice (yellowing of the skin or eyes), abdominal swelling, or severe headaches could point to organ damage, particularly to the liver, kidneys, or brain, caused by prolonged substance use.

6. **Inability to stop or control physical health decline:** Being unable to stop using substances despite ongoing damage to your body highlights the need for professional help. Addiction often leads to escalating health problems, and specialised treatment is necessary to halt or reverse the damage.

7. **Persistent or worsening physical symptoms:** Pain, dizziness, or shortness of breath that persists or worsens over time should prompt consultation with a healthcare provider. These signs may indicate serious conditions such as

cardiovascular disease, lung disease, or gastrointestinal problems linked to addiction.

8. **Concern from medical professionals or loved ones:** Concerns expressed by doctors or loved ones about your physical health due to substance use may highlight significant health risks. Sometimes, the physical damage caused by addiction is more apparent to others, and early intervention can help prevent further harm.

Recognising when addiction is impacting your physical health is crucial. The sooner you seek help, the better the chances of preventing long-term damage. With the right support, many physical effects can be managed or reversed, leading to improved health and a better quality of life. Don't wait – take action now for a healthier future.

My personal experience

Burnout took a toll on my physical health in ways I couldn't initially see. My energy levels were almost non-existent, my sleep patterns were constantly disrupted, and my body felt sluggish. As I worked towards a reset, I began to recognise how these physical symptoms were manifestations of the burnout itself. Taking care of my body became a key part of my recovery. I learned that physical health was not just about eliminating harmful behaviours; it was about nourishing my body with what it needed to restore balance.

Conclusion

The connection between addiction and physical health is both profound and complex. Addiction does not only affect the mind – it leaves an indelible mark on the body. Whether through direct damage to organs and bodily systems or through the neglect of essential healthcare, the physical consequences of addiction can be long-lasting and sometimes irreversible.

Recognising the importance of this connection is vital for both treatment and prevention. Early intervention, medical care, and lifestyle changes can significantly improve outcomes for individuals grappling with addiction. By addressing both the psychological and physical aspects of addiction, it becomes possible not only to break free from the cycle of dependency but also to restore health and wellbeing for a better, more fulfilling life.

CHAPTER 12

THE CONNECTION BETWEEN ADDICTION AND MENTAL WELLBEING

Addiction and mental wellbeing are deeply interconnected, often existing in a complex, cyclical relationship. Understanding this connection is essential for addressing both issues effectively. This chapter explores the link between addiction and mental health, how they influence each other, and why they often occur together. It also outlines steps for addressing these issues, providing a pathway towards healing and recovery. Subsequent chapters in this section of the book look at the relationship between addiction and specific mental health issues.

The connection between mental wellbeing and addiction

The relationship between addiction and mental wellbeing is bidirectional: poor mental health can increase the risk of addiction, while addiction can worsen or contribute to the onset of mental health problems. Many individuals with mental health challenges, such as anxiety, depression, or trauma, turn to substances or addictive behaviours as a form of self-medication to manage emotional pain. However, this reliance can quickly spiral into addiction, creating a vicious cycle as the addiction worsens mental health symptoms. Conversely, addiction itself can trigger or intensify mental health issues, as substances disrupt brain chemistry and behaviours associated with addiction lead to feelings of guilt, shame, and isolation. Understanding this interplay is critical for effective treatment, as addressing both addiction and underlying mental health conditions simultaneously offers the best path to recovery.

Mental wellbeing – a complex balance

Mental wellbeing is not just the absence of mental illness; it is a state of positive mental health. It encompasses emotional, psychological, and social wellbeing, affecting how we think, feel, and act. Good mental wellbeing allows individuals to cope with stress, maintain healthy relationships, and make decisions that promote a meaningful life. Conversely, poor mental health can lead to conditions like depression, anxiety, and other mental health disorders.

How mental health problems can lead to addiction

One of the primary reasons individuals turn to addictive substances or behaviours is as a form of self-medication. People experiencing mental health challenges such as anxiety, depression, or trauma often use drugs, alcohol, or other addictive behaviours to numb emotional pain, reduce stress, or escape overwhelming thoughts.

However, what begins as an attempt to manage distress can quickly spiral into dependence. The relief that substances or behaviours offer is temporary, leading to repeated use to maintain that fleeting sense of calm or happiness. Over time, this coping mechanism becomes an addiction, with the brain becoming reliant on external substances to regulate emotions.

How addiction can lead to mental health problems

On the other side of the equation, addiction itself can precipitate mental health issues. Substance abuse can disrupt brain chemistry, impairing the regulation of mood and cognition. For instance, excessive alcohol or drug use can lead to anxiety, depression, or paranoia. Behavioural addictions, such as gambling or excessive gaming, can lead to feelings of guilt, shame, and isolation, further contributing to mental health problems.

Moreover, the lifestyle associated with addiction - financial strain, damaged relationships, loss of employment, and social isolation - can intensify feelings of hopelessness and despair, fuelling mental health struggles. This creates a vicious cycle where addiction exacerbates mental health issues, which in turn drive further addictive behaviour.

Understanding the connection between addiction and mental health

Understanding the relationship between addiction and mental health is crucial for developing effective, integrated treatment plans that address both conditions simultaneously. When addiction and mental health challenges are treated in isolation, the root causes or contributing factors of one may be overlooked, increasing the risk of relapse or incomplete recovery.

1. **Biological factors:** Biology plays a significant role in the connection between addiction and mental wellbeing. Neurotransmitters, such as dopamine and serotonin, are crucial for regulating mood and pleasure. Addiction disrupts these neurotransmitters, leading to mood disorders like anxiety and depression. Genetic make-up also has a role; statistics show that individuals with a family history of

mental illness or addiction are more susceptible to developing both conditions.

2. **Psychological factors:** Psychological factors are central to the link between addiction and mental health. Trauma, stress, and unresolved emotional issues increase vulnerability to both addiction and mental health problems. People with low self-esteem or poor coping skills, or those exposed to long-term stressors, are at higher risk of seeking relief through addictive substances or behaviours, which in turn may damage their mental health further.

3. **Social and environmental factors:** Social and environmental influences also impact the relationship between addiction and mental wellbeing. Poverty, social isolation, and exposure to high-stress environments can trigger both mental health issues and addictive behaviours. In addition, cultural attitudes towards substances and behavioural addictions can normalise or exacerbate the connection. For instance, in some environments, binge-drinking is socially accepted, which can make individuals more susceptible to addiction and its mental health impacts.

How to break the cycle

Breaking the cycle of addiction and mental health problems contributing to one another requires treating both issues together. Addressing them separately can lead to relapse and worsening symptoms. A combined approach offers the best chance for recovery, providing the support needed for lasting healing.

1. **Seek professional help:** Integrated treatment – where both addiction and mental health are treated concurrently – is essential. Mental health professionals, addiction

counsellors, and medical practitioners can work together to develop a treatment plan that addresses the complexities of both conditions. Cognitive behavioural therapy (CBT), dialectical behaviour therapy (DBT), and other therapeutic approaches can help individuals identify and manage the root causes of their addiction and mental health challenges. (See 'When to seek help' below.)

2. **Build a support network:** Support from friends, family, or support groups can be crucial in recovery. Groups such as Alcoholics Anonymous (AA), Narcotics Anonymous (NA), and other addiction support groups can provide a safe space to share experiences and find encouragement from others who understand the struggle. Similarly, mental health support groups offer community and guidance for managing conditions like anxiety or depression.

3. **Focus on self-care and mindfulness:** Self-care is a critical component of maintaining mental wellbeing and preventing relapse into addiction. Engaging in healthy activities such as exercise, meditation, and creative hobbies can help regulate emotions and reduce the temptation to rely on addictive substances or behaviours. Mindfulness practices, in particular, can be transformative. By staying present in the moment, individuals can become more aware of their thoughts and feelings, reducing the impulse to escape through addiction.

4. **Address underlying trauma:** For many, unresolved trauma is at the heart of the addiction-mental health cycle. Trauma-informed therapy, such as eye movement desensitisation and reprocessing (EMDR), or somatic experiencing, can help individuals process and heal from past traumas, thereby reducing the need to self-medicate

through addictive behaviours.

5. **Develop healthy coping mechanisms:** One of the most effective ways to break the addiction-mental health connection is to replace destructive behaviours with healthy coping mechanisms. Developing better stress management techniques, such as deep breathing, journaling, or engaging in physical activities, can provide healthier alternatives to addiction. These skills are often cultivated in therapy; however, they can be practised daily to reinforce positive mental health.

When to seek help

Recognising when to seek help for mental health challenges is crucial for early intervention and effective treatment. Mental health issues can often go unnoticed or untreated, leading to further complications. Understanding the signs that indicate professional support is needed can help individuals take the first step towards recovery and better wellbeing.

1. **Persistent feelings of sadness or anxiety:** If feelings of sadness, worry, or hopelessness persist for weeks or months and begin to interfere with daily life, it may be time to seek help. Prolonged emotional distress can indicate conditions like depression or anxiety disorders, which benefit greatly from professional support.

2. **Difficulty managing daily responsibilities:** When mental health challenges make it difficult to fulfil responsibilities at work, school, or home, seeking help is essential. Struggling to manage daily tasks can signal worsening symptoms that, if left untreated, may significantly impact overall wellbeing.

3. **Changes in sleep or appetite:** Significant changes in sleep patterns, such as insomnia or excessive sleeping, or noticeable shifts in appetite, like overeating or loss of appetite, may indicate an underlying mental health issue. These symptoms often accompany conditions like depression or anxiety and warrant medical or psychological intervention.

4. **Withdrawal from social connections:** Withdrawing from friends, family, and social activities is a common sign of mental health decline. Isolation often exacerbates mental health issues, and seeking support can help prevent further emotional detachment and loneliness.

5. **Intrusive or harmful thoughts:** Persistent thoughts of self-harm, harming others, or overwhelming despair are serious indicators of a mental health crisis. Immediate help is necessary, as these thoughts often signal severe depression, anxiety, or suicidal ideation.

6. **Feeling overwhelmed by stress or trauma:** If stress or past traumatic events feel unmanageable and are negatively affecting your mental health, it is important to seek help. Left untreated, ongoing stress and unresolved trauma can lead to disorders like post-traumatic stress disorder (PTSD), requiring professional intervention to address and heal.

7. **Inability to cope with emotions or situations:** Struggling to cope with emotional distress or difficult situations, such as overwhelming anger or fear, is another sign that help is needed. These challenges can lead to emotional outbursts or strained relationships; however, therapy can provide tools to develop healthier coping strategies.

If any of these signs are present, it is essential to seek professional help as soon as possible. Early intervention can prevent the cycle from worsening and increase the likelihood of successful recovery.

Conclusion

The connection between addiction and mental wellbeing is undeniable and complex. Both issues feed into each other, often creating a cycle that is difficult to break without intervention. However, with the right support, it is possible to address both addiction and mental health challenges simultaneously. By seeking professional help, building a strong support network, focusing on self-care, and addressing underlying trauma, individuals can regain control of their lives and work towards lasting recovery.

This journey is neither quick nor easy, but it is possible. Understanding the connection between addiction and mental health is the first step in finding a path to a healthier, more balanced life.

CHAPTER 13

THE CONNECTION BETWEEN ADDICTION AND EMOTIONAL HEALTH

Addiction is far more than a physical dependency on substances or behaviours; it is deeply intertwined with our emotional world. Often driven by emotional pain, addiction can become a way to cope with overwhelming feelings, creating a powerful and damaging connection between emotional turmoil and addictive behaviours. This chapter explores the emotional foundations of addiction, why it develops, how it perpetuates itself, and, crucially, what can be done to break the emotional chains that bind individuals to their addictions.

The connection between emotional health and addiction

Addiction often stems from an attempt to manage emotional pain, such as stress, anxiety, trauma, or loneliness, offering temporary relief from these overwhelming feelings. However, as addiction takes hold, it exacerbates emotional distress, impairing the brain's ability to regulate emotions naturally and deepening feelings of shame, guilt, and isolation. This creates a destructive loop where emotional suffering fuels addiction, and addiction worsens emotional health.

Addressing this connection is essential for recovery, as healing requires not only overcoming the addiction; it is also confronting and processing the underlying emotional issues that sustain it.

The emotional roots of addiction

At the heart of addiction lies a struggle with unresolved emotional pain. People often turn to addictive substances or behaviours as a means of escaping or dulling painful emotions, whether they stem from trauma, stress, loneliness, or other deep-seated feelings. When faced with emotional distress, the temporary relief provided by alcohol, drugs, gambling, or even compulsive behaviours like shopping or eating can seem like a lifeline. However, this reliance on external substances or actions to manage emotions often deepens the emotional wounds it was meant to heal.

For many, addiction begins as an emotional crutch. Feelings of anxiety, depression, anger, or emptiness can feel unbearable, and addiction offers a way to suppress or distract from these difficult emotions. The relief, however, is fleeting. Over time, as the addiction takes hold, individuals find themselves more emotionally vulnerable, with their ability to cope with life's challenges severely diminished. The emotional connection to addiction becomes a self-perpetuating cycle, where addiction exacerbates the very emotions it was meant to relieve.

How emotions drive addiction

Emotions are a key driver of addiction, especially when they are overwhelming. Many turn to substances or behaviours to cope with feelings like stress, anxiety, or depression. While addiction provides temporary relief, it creates a cycle that worsens emotional pain and deepens the dependency. Here's how it unfolds:

1. **Escaping emotional pain:** One of the most common emotional triggers for addiction is the desire to escape. People may use substances like alcohol or drugs, or engage in behaviours like gambling or binge eating, as a way to numb their emotional pain. Whether it's past trauma, feelings of inadequacy, or everyday stress, these emotions can feel insurmountable, and addiction offers a temporary reprieve.

2. **Emotionally charged cravings:** Addiction is not just about physical cravings; emotional cravings often drive the need for the substance or behaviour. For instance, someone may crave alcohol not because they are physically dependent, but because they associate drinking with emotional release or comfort during times of sadness or frustration. These emotional cravings can be just as powerful, if not more so, than the physical ones.

3. **Emotional dysregulation:** As addiction progresses, it interferes with the brain's ability to regulate emotions naturally. The brain becomes reliant on the addictive substance or behaviour to release dopamine, a chemical that plays a role in feelings of pleasure and reward. Without the addictive trigger, the brain struggles to manage emotions effectively, leading to heightened anxiety, irritability, or depression when the individual is not engaging in the addictive behaviour.

4. **Reinforcing negative emotions:** Addiction can fuel negative emotions like guilt, shame, and hopelessness. People trapped in addiction often feel a profound sense of failure, unable to break free from their behaviour despite their best efforts. This emotional burden can reinforce the addictive cycle, as they turn once again to the very substance or behaviour that is causing their distress.

5. **Emotional isolation:** Addiction can cause a person to withdraw from relationships and social connections, either out of shame or because their behaviour has led to conflict with loved ones. This isolation can deepen feelings of loneliness and depression, both of which are major contributors to emotional health issues. Emotional isolation reinforces the addiction, as individuals may feel they have nowhere to turn for emotional support.

How addiction and emotions are linked

Addiction and emotions are closely linked because emotional pain often drives addictive behaviours. Addiction also disrupts emotional regulation, making it harder to cope with feelings, which deepens dependency. Understanding this connection is key to addressing addiction's emotional aspects.

1. **Self-medication:** A common explanation for why addiction takes hold is the concept of self-medication. Individuals often use substances or behaviours to 'treat' their emotional pain. For example, someone dealing with anxiety might use alcohol to calm their nerves, or a person facing depression may use drugs to feel temporarily uplifted. Unfortunately, while these methods may provide short-term relief, they come with long-term emotional costs. As the addiction grows, so does the emotional toll, creating a cycle of dependency.

2. **Impact on brain chemistry:** Addiction changes the brain's chemistry, especially in areas related to emotion regulation. Over time, the brain's ability to manage stress, anxiety, and other emotions without the aid of addictive substances or behaviours is diminished. This makes it even harder for

people to cope with their emotions, driving them further into their addiction to maintain emotional balance.

3. **Emotional trauma:** For many, addiction is rooted in past emotional trauma. Unresolved emotional wounds - whether from childhood abuse, neglect, or other traumatic experiences - can drive people towards addiction as a way to manage or suppress their pain. These individuals often lack the emotional tools to process their trauma, leading them to seek comfort in destructive ways.

4. **Emotional vulnerability:** Some individuals are more emotionally vulnerable than others, whether due to genetics, upbringing, or life experiences. This emotional sensitivity can make them more susceptible to addiction, as they seek ways to soothe their intense emotional experiences. The connection between heightened emotional sensitivity and addiction is well-established, with many people finding it harder to cope with life's emotional ups and downs without turning to addictive behaviours.

Breaking the emotional cycle of addiction

Understanding the emotional connection to addiction is the first step in breaking the cycle. The key to recovery lies in addressing not only the addiction itself but also the underlying emotional pain that drives it. Here are some strategies that focus on healing the emotional aspect of addiction:

1. **Develop emotional awareness:** One of the most important steps in overcoming addiction is developing emotional awareness. Many individuals trapped in addiction have spent years numbing their emotions, to the point where they may struggle to recognise or understand what they're

feeling. Practices such as mindfulness, meditation, or journaling can help individuals reconnect with their emotions and begin to identify what triggers their addictive behaviours.

2. **Therapeutic intervention:** Professional help is often necessary to address both the addiction and the emotional issues that underpin it. Therapy, particularly approaches like cognitive behavioural therapy (CBT) or dialectical behaviour therapy (DBT), can help individuals understand the emotional roots of their addiction and develop healthier ways to cope with their feelings. Working through past traumas, grief, or unresolved emotional conflicts is crucial in creating lasting emotional stability.

3. **Building emotional resilience:** Emotional resilience refers to the ability to handle stress and emotional challenges without resorting to addictive behaviours. Building this resilience is vital for breaking the emotional cycle of addiction. Developing healthy coping mechanisms - such as exercise, creative expression, or talking with supportive friends - can help individuals manage emotional difficulties without turning to addiction.

4. **Addressing emotional triggers:** Identifying and addressing emotional triggers is key to preventing relapse. Emotional triggers are situations, feelings, or thoughts that lead to cravings for the addictive substance or behaviour. These can include stress, boredom, anger, or sadness. Learning to recognise and cope with these triggers in a healthier way can reduce the emotional drive toward addiction.

5. **Building emotional support networks:** Addiction often thrives in isolation, where emotional pain can go unchecked.

Building a strong support network - whether through friends, family, or support groups - can provide a crucial outlet for dealing with emotional struggles. Being able to talk openly about emotions with trusted individuals can help to reduce feelings of isolation and emotional burden.

6. **Address emotional trauma:** For those whose addiction is rooted in past trauma, healing these emotional wounds is essential for long-term recovery. Trauma-focused therapies, such as eye movement desensitisation and reprocessing (EMDR), or trauma-informed cognitive therapy, can help individuals process and heal from past traumas. Addressing the emotional pain that drives addiction is crucial for breaking the cycle and improving emotional health.

When to seek help

Recognising when addiction has begun to negatively affect emotional health is a crucial step towards recovery. If emotional struggles become overwhelming and persistent, or if addictive behaviours are increasingly relied upon to cope with emotions, it's essential to reach out for support. Seeking help early can prevent the emotional damage from deepening and help break the cycle of addiction. Here are key signs that it may be time to seek professional help:

1. **Overwhelming emotional distress:** When emotions like anxiety, depression, anger, or sadness become difficult to manage or persist over time, it indicates that emotional health is being compromised by addiction. These emotions can grow increasingly intense and unmanageable, interfering with daily life.

2. **Reliance on addiction to cope:** If addictive substances

or behaviours are being used more frequently to escape or numb emotions, this signifies that emotional health is deteriorating. Addiction becomes a way to avoid facing underlying emotional pain, leading to further emotional and psychological harm.

3. **Failed attempts to manage or quit:** Repeatedly trying to control or quit addictive behaviours without success can be a sign that the emotional health issues driving the addiction have not been properly addressed. This can lead to feelings of hopelessness, frustration, and self-blame, all of which worsen emotional health.

4. **Worsening emotional health despite efforts:** If emotional health continues to decline despite efforts to address it, it may be time to seek professional intervention. Addiction often feeds emotional instability, and without proper treatment, emotional distress can spiral out of control.

5. **Loss of emotional connection and isolation:** Addiction can lead to emotional isolation, where a person feels cut off from relationships or support systems. If you begin withdrawing from others due to shame or guilt, or feel emotionally distant and disconnected, it's important to seek help to restore these connections and improve emotional wellbeing.

Recognising these signs early and seeking the right support can be the first step in breaking the destructive cycle of addiction and emotional distress.

My personal experience

With so much going on in my life at the time when I needed to reset, emotionally I felt flat; there was nothing left. I couldn't even speak. I had hit the floor, and I was still trying to get up. The exhaustion masked my true feelings, making it difficult to identify what I needed or how to express it. Part of my reset involved learning to sit with my feelings, however uncomfortable. That space for emotional honesty became the foundation for rebuilding resilience.

Conclusion

Addiction and emotional pain are deeply intertwined. For many individuals, addiction begins as an attempt to manage or escape from overwhelming emotions, although it quickly becomes a trap that deepens emotional suffering. Breaking free from addiction requires not only addressing the physical aspects of dependency; it is also healing the emotional wounds that drive it. By focusing on emotional awareness, developing resilience, and seeking support, individuals can begin the journey towards emotional healing and long-term recovery from addiction. The journey may be challenging; however, with a deep understanding of the emotional roots of addiction, recovery is possible.

CHAPTER 14

THE CONNECTION BETWEEN ADDICTION AND SPIRITUAL WELLBEING

Addiction is not solely a physical or psychological battle; it also has profound implications for the soul. When individuals struggle with addiction, they often find themselves disconnected - not just from others or from reality, but from a deeper sense of purpose, meaning, and spiritual wellbeing. The concept of spiritual wellbeing transcends religious belief; it speaks to our sense of inner peace, connection, and alignment with our values. This chapter explores the deep and complex relationship between addiction and spiritual wellbeing, examining why this connection exists, what makes it happen, and how a spiritual approach can offer a pathway to recovery. We will also explore when and how to nurture spiritual wellbeing as a means of preventing or healing from addiction.

The connection between spiritual wellbeing and addiction

Addiction often stems from a sense of emptiness or disconnection, driving individuals to seek external substances or behaviours for relief. In contrast, spiritual wellbeing provides inner peace and a sense of purpose, offering a deeper fulfilment that addiction cannot. By addressing the spiritual void underlying addiction, individuals can reconnect with their true selves and embark on a path to healing and recovery.

How addiction and spiritual wellbeing are connected

Understanding the link between addiction and spiritual wellbeing sheds light on the emotional void that often drives addictive behaviours. This section examines the spiritual aspects of addiction and the quest for deeper meaning.

1. **The human search for meaning:** At its core, addiction often arises from a deep void or disconnection in an individual's life. Many people who suffer from addiction describe a sense of emptiness or meaninglessness, which they attempt to fill with substances or behaviours. This search for something beyond the physical - for meaning, purpose, or a deeper connection - is a spiritual need. When this need goes unmet, it can manifest in the compulsive seeking of external satisfaction, whether through alcohol, drugs, gambling, or other forms of addiction.

2. **Disconnection from the self:** Addiction can be seen as a form of disconnection – from the self, from others, and from the world. Spiritual wellbeing, on the other hand, is about feeling connected to oneself, to one's values, and to a higher purpose. The deeper someone falls into addiction, the more they feel separated from their true self. This loss of identity and self-worth often exacerbates feelings of shame and hopelessness, making the cycle of addiction even more difficult to break.

3. **Spiritual crisis as a catalyst:** Many people experience

what is known as a 'spiritual crisis' - a period of existential questioning or emotional turbulence, where they begin to doubt the meaning of life, their purpose, or their connection to something greater. In response to this spiritual crisis, individuals may turn to substances or behaviours in an attempt to numb the discomfort. Unfortunately, this often leads them further away from the spiritual answers they are seeking, trapping them in a cycle of addiction and disconnection.

How addiction erodes spiritual wellbeing

Addiction erodes spiritual wellbeing by fostering isolation and self-destructive behaviours. This section delves into the mechanisms through which addiction disrupts the connection to one's spirit.

1. **Isolation and alienation:** Addiction thrives on isolation. As individuals become more consumed by their addictive behaviours, they often withdraw from social circles, family, and even their own values. This isolation leads to a sense of alienation - not just from other people, but from their own spiritual essence. Addiction replaces the pursuit of connection, peace, and meaning with temporary highs, leading to a growing sense of emptiness.

2. **Ego and control:** Addiction can be driven by an overwhelming need for control - over one's feelings, one's environment, and even one's spiritual journey. This need for control is antithetical to spiritual wellbeing, which often involves surrender, acceptance, and trust in something greater than oneself. The more individuals attempt to control their environment through addiction, the further they stray from spiritual growth.

3. **Self-destructive patterns:** At its core, addiction is often self-destructive. It is an attempt to fill a void with something that ultimately harms rather than heals. Spiritual wellbeing, by contrast, is about growth, compassion, and nurturing oneself. Addiction turns one against oneself, leading to shame, guilt, and further spiritual depletion.

What makes this connection so powerful

The relationship between addiction and spiritual wellbeing is powerful because both are rooted in the human need for fulfilment and connection. Addiction is often an attempt to find solace, peace, or relief from suffering. While it may provide temporary relief, it ultimately deepens the individual's spiritual disconnection. On the other hand, spiritual wellbeing offers a more profound and lasting sense of fulfilment by connecting individuals to their true selves and to a higher purpose.

1. **Addiction as a misguided search for spiritual fulfilment:** Many people who turn to addictive substances or behaviours are, consciously or unconsciously, searching for something greater. Whether it's a sense of belonging, inner peace, or a higher state of consciousness, addiction often starts as a way to fill this void. However, because it addresses only the physical or emotional aspects of the problem, addiction can never fully meet these deeper spiritual needs.

2. **Spiritual wellbeing as a foundation for recovery:** Recovery from addiction requires more than just physical detoxification; it requires a holistic approach that addresses the mind, body, and spirit. For many people, the process of reconnecting with their spiritual wellbeing becomes a vital component of healing. It offers them a sense of purpose,

hope, and inner strength, which helps them resist the pull of addiction.

3. **The power of acceptance and surrender:** One of the key principles in many spiritual traditions is the concept of surrender – the idea of letting go of the need to control everything and trusting in a higher power or greater purpose. This principle is also central to many addiction recovery programmes, such as Alcoholics Anonymous, which encourage individuals to acknowledge their powerlessness over addiction and surrender to a higher power, however they define it. This spiritual surrender can help individuals break free from the obsessive need to control their addiction, leading to lasting recovery.

How to rebuild spiritual wellbeing in the context of addiction

Rebuilding spiritual wellbeing in recovery is essential for lasting healing. This section offers practical strategies for reconnecting with one's spirit and fostering a sense of purpose.

1. **Practising mindfulness and meditation:** One of the most effective ways to reconnect with spiritual wellbeing is through mindfulness and meditation. These practices allow individuals to quiet their minds, tune in to their inner selves, and experience a sense of peace that is not reliant on external substances or behaviours. Regular mindfulness or meditation can help individuals break the cycle of addiction by offering them an alternative way to cope with stress, cravings, and emotional turmoil.

2. **Exploring spiritual practices:** For those in recovery, exploring different spiritual practices can be a powerful way

to restore a sense of purpose and connection. This could include prayer, yoga, journaling, or attending spiritual gatherings. These practices don't have to be tied to a specific religion; they can simply be ways to cultivate inner peace and a deeper connection to something greater than oneself.

3. **Engaging in acts of service:** Spiritual wellbeing is often nurtured through acts of compassion and service to others. Volunteering, helping those in need, or simply being kind and present for others, can help individuals feel more connected to the world around them. These acts of service remind us of the interconnectedness of all life and can provide a sense of fulfilment and purpose that addiction cannot.

4. **Forgiveness and self-compassion:** Addiction often comes with a heavy burden of guilt, shame, and self-judgement. Healing spiritually involves practising forgiveness - both of oneself and of others. By cultivating self-compassion, individuals can begin to heal the emotional and spiritual wounds that drive their addiction. This can be achieved through therapy, spiritual guidance, or simply adopting a more compassionate mindset towards oneself.

5. **Seeking community and support:** Spiritual wellbeing often flourishes in community. Whether it's through a recovery group, a spiritual organisation, or a supportive group of friends, surrounding oneself with like-minded individuals who value spiritual growth can be incredibly healing. These communities offer connection, support, and encouragement, helping individuals feel less isolated in their journey towards recovery.

When to focus on spiritual wellbeing in addiction recovery

Identifying key moments in the recovery process to emphasise spiritual wellbeing can enhance resilience and success. This section discusses specific times when focusing on spirituality is particularly beneficial.

1. **During early recovery:** The early stages of recovery from addiction can be physically and emotionally intense. While the focus may initially be on physical detox and stabilising mental health, it is also crucial to begin nurturing spiritual wellbeing during this period. Early recovery is a time when individuals often feel lost or disconnected, making it the ideal moment to introduce spiritual practices that can help them regain a sense of purpose and connection.

2. **When facing relapse:** Relapse is a common part of the recovery process, and it often occurs when individuals feel overwhelmed or disconnected from their recovery goals. When the threat of relapse looms, it is important to turn to spiritual practices as a way of reconnecting with one's deeper values and purpose. Mindfulness, meditation, and community support can all help individuals regain their sense of inner strength and resist the urge to return to addictive behaviours.

3. **When seeking long-term recovery:** Long-term recovery from addiction requires ongoing commitment and self-awareness. As individuals move further along their recovery journey, nurturing spiritual wellbeing becomes an essential part of maintaining sobriety and inner peace. Regular spiritual practices, acts of service, and self-reflection

can help individuals stay grounded and focused on their long-term goals.

When to seek help

Spiritual wellbeing plays a vital role in recovery from addiction, and recognising when to seek help can be crucial in maintaining or restoring inner peace. The following situations highlight when spiritual support is particularly beneficial, offering a pathway to healing and reconnection with one's deeper sense of purpose.

1. **Feelings of spiritual emptiness or disconnection:** When individuals experience a profound sense of emptiness or a lack of connection to something greater than themselves, it may signal the need for spiritual guidance. This disconnection can contribute to feelings of despair, which may fuel addictive behaviours. Seeking help can aid the restoration of a sense of meaning and alignment with personal values.

2. **Struggling with existential questions:** If you are grappling with questions about life's purpose or feel lost in your journey, turning to spiritual support can offer clarity. These questions often arise in moments of crisis or in the midst of addiction, and spiritual practices can provide the insights needed to navigate them.

3. **Experiencing a spiritual crisis:** A spiritual crisis, characterised by intense doubt or loss of faith, can make recovery from addiction more challenging. Seeking spiritual help during such a time can help in rediscovering a sense of hope, peace, and trust in a higher power or purpose, which is crucial for healing.

4. **Feeling overwhelmed by guilt and shame:** Addiction often brings a heavy burden of guilt and shame, which can damage one's spiritual wellbeing. When these feelings become overwhelming, it may be time to seek support from a spiritual guide or community, where forgiveness, compassion, and healing can be nurtured.

5. **Inability to find inner peace or acceptance:** If you are struggling to find inner peace or are resistant to accepting your current reality, spiritual practices like mindfulness, meditation, or prayer can be instrumental in developing a deeper sense of acceptance and serenity. Seeking help can guide you towards practices that help release control and foster spiritual surrender.

6. **Facing the threat of relapse:** When the temptation to return to addictive behaviours becomes strong, reconnecting with spiritual practices can provide the strength needed to resist. Seeking help from a spiritual community or mentor during these moments can provide guidance, support, and the spiritual tools needed to maintain recovery.

By addressing spiritual needs and nurturing inner peace, individuals can find strength, purpose, and a deeper connection to themselves and the world around them. Recognising when to seek help is an important part of reclaiming spiritual wellbeing and breaking free from the cycle of addiction, ultimately leading to a more fulfilling and meaningful life.

My personal experience

I have always believed there is far more to this world than what we can see. Whether one calls it spirituality, religion, energy, or something else entirely is a personal choice. What matters is the belief in something greater – a presence or force far beyond the individual, one that holds a deeper awareness of the whole. Something that sees all, knows all, and moves through everything. When we surrender our life to this greater power, we release the weight of fear, stress, and worry. We begin to live with the understanding that everything – past, present, and future – unfolds with purpose. Believe, and let go.

Conclusion

The connection between addiction and spiritual wellbeing is deep and profound. Addiction often arises from a disconnection from one's true self, values, and purpose, while spiritual wellbeing offers a pathway to healing and reconnection. By nurturing spiritual practices, engaging in acts of service, and fostering self-compassion, individuals can find a sense of peace and fulfilment that addiction cannot provide. Recovery from addiction is not just about breaking physical dependencies; it is about rediscovering the deeper, spiritual aspects of life that provide true meaning and purpose. Through this journey, individuals can heal not only their bodies and minds; they can also heal their souls.

CHAPTER 15

THE CONNECTION BETWEEN ADDICTION AND LACK OF SLEEP

In the intricate web of factors that contribute to addiction, one often overlooked element is sleep. The relationship between sleep and addiction is not only strong; it is also cyclical, with each influencing the other in profound ways. In this chapter, we explore how lack of sleep can fuel addictive behaviours, why this connection exists, and what steps can be taken to break this destructive cycle.

The connection between lack of sleep and addiction

Sleep deprivation impairs the brain's ability to regulate emotions, make decisions, and control impulses, increasing vulnerability to addictive behaviours. It also disrupts the brain's reward system, reducing dopamine sensitivity and driving individuals to seek artificial boosts through substances or behaviours. Conversely, addiction often leads to sleep disturbances, whether through the stimulating effects of substances, withdrawal symptoms, or psychological distress. This creates a vicious cycle: poor sleep fosters addiction, and addiction perpetuates poor sleep. Breaking this loop requires addressing both issues simultaneously, prioritising sleep as a key component of recovery.

The importance of sleep

Sleep is not a luxury; it is a biological necessity. It plays a critical role in cognitive function, emotional regulation, memory consolidation, and overall mental health. Adults typically need seven to nine hours of sleep per night to function at their best. Chronic sleep deprivation can impair decision-making, increase impulsivity, and reduce emotional resilience, all of which are key factors in addiction.

For those struggling with addiction or in recovery, sleep disturbances are common. The reasons for this are complex, involving physiological, psychological, and behavioural components. Sleep problems can both exacerbate addiction and be a consequence of it, creating a vicious cycle that is difficult to break.

How lack of sleep contributes to addiction

Lack of sleep plays a crucial role in addiction by impairing brain function, decision-making, and emotional regulation. This creates a cycle where sleep deprivation and addiction reinforce each other, making recovery more difficult. Here's how sleep deprivation fuels addiction:

1. **Impaired cognitive function and decision-making:** Sleep is essential for the brain's ability to process information and make sound decisions. When sleep-deprived, the brain struggles to weigh risks and rewards properly. This cognitive impairment can lower an individual's ability to resist addictive substances or behaviours. It weakens the prefrontal cortex, which is responsible for self-control, making impulsive decisions more likely.

2. **Increased stress and anxiety:** A lack of sleep elevates stress hormones like cortisol. Over time, this chronic stress can

lead to heightened anxiety, a common trigger for addictive behaviour. Substances like alcohol, nicotine, or drugs often become coping mechanisms for dealing with stress, further deepening the addiction.

3. **Reward system dysregulation:** Sleep deprivation affects the brain's reward system by altering dopamine levels, the chemical responsible for feelings of pleasure and reward. In a sleep-deprived state, the brain seeks out artificial ways to boost dopamine production, making addictive substances or behaviours more appealing. This is why many people find themselves craving sugar, caffeine, or even stronger substances when they are tired.

4. **Mood and emotional instability:** Sleep is vital for emotional regulation. A lack of it can lead to irritability, mood swings, and depression. Negative emotional states often drive people to seek relief through substances or addictive behaviours. This emotional instability also diminishes motivation, which can derail recovery efforts for those trying to overcome addiction.

5. **Physical and mental fatigue:** Physical fatigue caused by lack of sleep can weaken the body's natural defences against stress and anxiety. Mental exhaustion can make it harder to engage in the self-discipline needed to resist cravings or adhere to recovery programmes. This exhaustion can make the prospect of using substances seem like an easy escape.

How the connection happens

The connection between sleep and addiction can be traced to the brain's chemistry and structure. The body's circadian rhythms, which regulate the sleep-wake cycle, are controlled by areas in the brain that also manage emotions, memory, and impulse control. These same brain regions are heavily involved in addictive behaviours.

1. **Dopamine and the reward circuit:** Addiction and sleep deprivation both target the brain's reward circuit. Sleep loss reduces the sensitivity of this circuit, leading to a diminished ability to experience pleasure from natural rewards like social interactions or physical activity. To compensate, individuals may turn to addictive substances or behaviours that give an artificial dopamine boost.

2. **Stress response:** The brain's response to stress is heightened when sleep is lacking. Addiction often develops as a coping mechanism for dealing with stress and emotional pain. Without adequate sleep, the body is in a state of constant low-level stress, increasing vulnerability to addiction.

3. **Psychological factors:** Insomnia and other sleep disturbances are commonly associated with mental health disorders, such as anxiety and depression, both of which are risk factors for addiction. The psychological toll of sleep deprivation can push individuals towards substance use as a way to alleviate emotional distress.

4. **Circadian rhythm disruptions:** Irregular sleep patterns, such as those caused by shift work, travel, or chronic insomnia, disrupt the body's natural circadian rhythms. This misalignment can lead to increased cravings for substances and hinder the body's ability to manage stress, further fuelling addiction.

What to do

Improving sleep quality can be a critical component in both preventing addiction and supporting recovery. By prioritising sleep, individuals can strengthen their ability to resist addictive behaviours and promote overall mental and physical health.

1. **Establish a consistent sleep routine:** Going to bed and waking up at the same time every day helps regulate your body's internal clock, making it easier to fall asleep and wake up naturally. Avoid naps during the day, as they can interfere with night-time sleep.

2. **Create a sleep-friendly environment:** Your bedroom should be a quiet, dark, and cool space dedicated to sleep. Minimise noise, invest in comfortable bedding, and eliminate sources of bright light such as electronic devices.

3. **Limit stimulants:** Caffeine, nicotine, and other stimulants interfere with the ability to fall asleep. Avoid consuming these substances in the afternoon and evening. If possible, eliminate them altogether, as they can contribute to both sleep problems and addiction.

4. **Mindfulness and relaxation techniques:** Practising mindfulness, meditation, or deep-breathing exercises before bed can help reduce stress and anxiety, making it easier to fall asleep. These techniques can also be useful during the day to combat the urge to use addictive substances.

5. **Exercise regularly:** Physical activity promotes better sleep and reduces stress. However, it's important to avoid vigorous exercise close to bedtime, as it can increase alertness and make it harder to sleep.

6. **Seek professional help:** If sleep problems persist, it may

be beneficial to consult a healthcare professional. Cognitive behavioural therapy for insomnia (CBT-I) is a proven treatment that can help those struggling with both sleep deprivation and addiction. Similarly, support from addiction specialists, psychologists, or sleep specialists may be necessary to break the cycle.

7. **Limit screen time:** Exposure to blue light from phones, computers, and televisions can interfere with your body's ability to produce melatonin, the hormone that signals it's time for sleep. Avoid screens for at least an hour before bed.

8. **Address underlying mental health issues:** Anxiety, depression, and other mental health issues can contribute to both sleep problems and addiction. Treating these conditions through therapy, medication, or lifestyle changes is essential for improving sleep and preventing relapse into addictive behaviours.

When to seek help

If you or someone you know is facing both addiction and sleep deprivation, it's essential to seek professional help as soon as possible. The combination of prolonged sleep loss and addiction can significantly hinder recovery, making it more difficult to break the cycle. Early intervention can help address both issues before they escalate. The following signs indicate that professional support may be needed:

1. **Chronic insomnia:** Difficulty falling asleep or staying asleep that persists for weeks or months can significantly affect physical and mental health. If sleep problems become persistent, professional intervention may be necessary to address the underlying causes, such as addiction or anxiety.

2. **Increased cravings for substances:** Sleep deprivation can heighten cravings for substances or addictive behaviours, often as a way of coping with fatigue or emotional distress. If the desire to use substances increases during periods of tiredness, it's crucial to seek help to manage both the addiction and the sleep issues.

3. **Difficulty concentrating, making decisions, or controlling impulses:** Sleep loss impairs cognitive function, making it harder to concentrate, think clearly, and make decisions. If these cognitive issues interfere with daily life and lead to impulsive behaviour, it may indicate a need for professional treatment to address both sleep disturbances and addiction.

4. **Growing dependence on substances to sleep or relax:** If an individual increasingly relies on alcohol, drugs, or other substances to fall asleep or unwind, it creates a dangerous cycle that reinforces both the addiction and the sleep deprivation. This dependence should be addressed by a healthcare provider or addiction specialist.

5. **Increased anxiety or depression alongside sleep problems:** Sleep deprivation can worsen mental health conditions like anxiety and depression, which in turn fuel addictive behaviour. If sleep problems are accompanied by heightened anxiety, mood swings, or feelings of depression, seeking help from a mental health professional is vital to breaking the cycle and restoring balance.

Recognising these signs early and seeking professional help is critical for managing the interwoven challenges of addiction and sleep deprivation. The sooner support is sought, the better the chances of regaining control over both sleep and addictive behaviours.

My personal experience

Overworking and stress, as well as having a young family, often disrupted my sleep, leaving me fatigued and less able to cope with the day-to-day challenges of life. I didn't realise how much sleep deprivation was affecting my overall wellbeing until I started to prioritise sleep and rest. Through this reset, I understood that sleep is not just a physical need – it's essential for emotional, mental, and physical recovery. As I worked towards healthier habits, I noticed how improving my sleep patterns supported my journey and helped me feel more resilient and focused.

Conclusion

The link between sleep and addiction is powerful yet often under-recognised. Lack of sleep can weaken the brain's ability to resist cravings, impair decision-making, and increase emotional distress, all of which can drive addictive behaviours. By improving sleep quality through consistent routines, stress management, and professional support, individuals can reduce their risk of addiction or enhance their recovery process.

Addressing sleep issues is not just an afterthought in addiction treatment; it should be a central focus. As this chapter has shown, sleep is fundamental to our wellbeing, and its role in addiction is significant. Prioritising rest is not only a step towards better health; it is also a key element in breaking free from the grip of addiction.

CHAPTER 16

THE CONNECTION BETWEEN ADDICTION AND ADHD

Attention-deficit hyperactivity disorder (ADHD) is a neurodevelopmental condition characterised by symptoms of inattention, hyperactivity, and impulsivity. Affecting both children and adults, ADHD influences various aspects of life, including academic and professional performance, social interactions, and personal relationships. One significant area of concern is the heightened risk of addiction among individuals with ADHD. Research indicates that people with ADHD are more likely to engage in substance abuse, develop addictive behaviours, and experience difficulties in recovery. This chapter explores the intricate connection between ADHD and addiction, delving into the mechanisms underlying this link, the factors that contribute to it, and evidence-based strategies for intervention and management.

The connection between ADHD and addiction

Individuals with ADHD are significantly more prone to developing addictions due to shared underlying factors such as impulsivity, a tendency to seek immediate gratification, and deficiencies in the brain's reward system, particularly involving dopamine regulation. Many turn to addictive substances or behaviours as a way to self-medicate, temporarily alleviating symptoms like restlessness, anxiety, or difficulty concentrating. However, this often leads to a cycle of dependency that exacerbates both conditions. Understanding this connection is crucial for effective treatment and prevention strategies tailored to address the unique challenges faced by individuals with ADHD.

Understanding ADHD and addiction

ADHD is more than just an inability to focus or sit still. It is a complex condition with roots in the brain's structure and function, often influenced by genetic, environmental, and neurobiological factors. Key symptoms include difficulty maintaining attention, hyperactive behaviour, and impulsive actions that can disrupt daily functioning.

Addiction, on the other hand, is a chronic disorder characterised by compulsive engagement in rewarding stimuli despite adverse consequences. It can manifest in various forms, such as substance abuse (alcohol, drugs), behavioural addictions (gambling, gaming), and digital addictions (internet, social media). The common thread across these types of addiction is the loss of control over behaviour, leading to detrimental impacts on an individual's health, relationships, and overall quality of life.

The overlap between ADHD and addiction is a growing area of research, highlighting the need for a comprehensive understanding of how these two conditions interact. This understanding is crucial for developing effective treatment strategies that address both ADHD and addictive behaviours simultaneously.

How and why there is a connection with ADHD

The relationship between ADHD and addiction is complex, influenced by neurobiological, psychological, and environmental factors. Understanding how these conditions intersect is vital for recognising the heightened vulnerability of individuals with ADHD to addiction. Exploring the mechanisms and traits that link them highlights the importance of targeted interventions.

1. **Neurobiological factors:** Both ADHD and addiction are linked to dysfunctions in the brain's reward system, particularly involving neurotransmitters such as dopamine. Individuals with ADHD often exhibit lower levels of dopamine, a neurotransmitter critical for experiencing pleasure and reward. This deficiency can lead them to seek out stimulating activities or substances that provide a temporary boost in dopamine levels, creating a cycle where the pursuit of immediate gratification overrides long-term consequences.

2. **Impulsivity and risk-taking:** Impulsivity is a hallmark of ADHD, significantly increasing the risk of engaging in addictive behaviours. The inability to delay gratification or control impulses can make it challenging for individuals with ADHD to resist the allure of immediate rewards provided by addictive substances or activities. This impulsivity often leads to risk-taking behaviours, further compounding the likelihood of addiction.

3. **Self-medication hypothesis:** Many individuals with ADHD turn to drugs or alcohol as a form of self-medication, seeking relief from symptoms such as restlessness, anxiety, and mood instability. Substances like nicotine, alcohol, and illicit drugs can temporarily alleviate these symptoms, creating a deceptive sense of relief. Unfortunately, this coping mechanism can lead to a cycle of dependence, where the individual becomes reliant on substances to manage their ADHD symptoms.

4. **Environmental and social factors:** The challenges faced by individuals with ADHD, such as academic struggles, social difficulties, and low self-esteem, can contribute to the development of addiction. These environmental stressors often lead to feelings of frustration and failure, pushing individuals to seek solace in addictive behaviours as a means of escape. Additionally, exposure to substance use within social circles can further increase the risk of addiction.

Why the connection matters

Understanding the link between ADHD and addiction is crucial for effective treatment. ADHD increases addiction risk due to impulsivity and poor self-regulation. Early intervention can prevent escalation and improve long-term wellbeing. Here's why this connection matters:

1. **Early intervention:** Recognising the heightened risk can lead to early intervention, potentially preventing the development of addiction in individuals with ADHD. By identifying at-risk individuals and providing support early on, it is possible to mitigate the likelihood of addiction.

2. **Tailored treatment**: Treatments for addiction can be more effective when they take into account the presence of ADHD. Addressing both conditions simultaneously rather than in isolation can lead to more comprehensive and effective treatment plans, improving the likelihood of successful recovery.

3. **Improved outcomes:** Comprehensive care that addresses the underlying ADHD can lead to better long-term outcomes for individuals struggling with addiction. By

managing ADHD symptoms effectively, individuals may experience reduced cravings and an improved ability to cope with stressors, ultimately enhancing their quality of life.

What to do

Effectively addressing ADHD and addiction requires a comprehensive approach tailored to individual needs. By implementing evidence-based interventions and support systems, individuals can manage their symptoms and reduce the risk of addiction.

1. **Integrated treatment approaches:** Effective treatment should integrate interventions for both ADHD and addiction. This might include behavioural therapy, medication management, and support groups that address both issues concurrently. A multidisciplinary approach can ensure that all aspects of an individual's health are considered.

2. **Medication management:** Medications such as stimulants (e.g., methylphenidate) and non-stimulants (e.g., atomoxetine) can be used to manage ADHD symptoms, potentially reducing the need for self-medication through substance abuse. When prescribing medications, healthcare providers should monitor for any potential interactions with substances.

3. **Cognitive behavioural therapy (CBT):** CBT is effective in treating both ADHD and addiction. This form of therapy helps individuals develop coping strategies, improve impulse control, and address dysfunctional thought patterns that contribute to addictive behaviours. By fostering healthier thought processes, CBT can empower individuals to make better choices.

4. **Psychoeducation:** Educating individuals and their families about the connection between ADHD and addiction can empower them to seek appropriate help and support. Understanding the link between these conditions can reduce stigma and encourage proactive measures for managing both.

5. **Support networks:** Building strong support networks, including family, friends, and professional counsellors, is essential for individuals managing both ADHD and addiction. These networks can provide encouragement, accountability, and a sense of community, helping individuals feel less isolated in their struggles.

When to seek help

Recognising the signs of unmanaged ADHD is crucial for preventing its escalation and ensuring that individuals receive the necessary support. Early intervention can reduce the impact of ADHD on daily life and prevent secondary issues, such as addiction or mental health problems, from developing. The following indicators suggest when it is time to seek professional help for ADHD:

1. **Persistent difficulty managing symptoms:** If ADHD symptoms - such as inattention, hyperactivity, or impulsivity - remain unmanageable despite medication or behavioural strategies, it may indicate that the current treatment plan needs adjustment or further evaluation.

2. **Increased struggles in key areas of life:** When ADHD symptoms significantly interfere with important areas of life, including work, school, or social relationships, seeking help can ensure the individual gets the support needed to navigate these challenges.

3. **Low self-esteem or frustration due to ADHD:** Persistent feelings of failure, frustration, or low self-worth related to ADHD symptoms may lead to emotional distress. Professional help can address these psychological effects and help individuals develop healthier coping mechanisms.

4. **Inability to control impulsive behaviours:** If impulsivity, a core symptom of ADHD, becomes difficult to control and leads to risky or harmful behaviours, professional intervention is crucial. This can include difficulties with spending, emotional outbursts, or engaging in other problematic actions.

Understanding when to seek help allows individuals with ADHD - and their families - to take proactive steps toward better management of the condition, improving overall quality of life and reducing the risk of developing co-occurring issues.

Conclusion

The connection between ADHD and addiction is complex yet well-documented. Understanding the neurobiological, psychological, and social factors that link these conditions is essential for effective intervention and treatment. By addressing both ADHD and addiction through integrated approaches, individuals can achieve better outcomes and lead healthier, more fulfilling lives. Early recognition and comprehensive care are key to breaking the cycle of addiction and managing ADHD effectively, paving the way for recovery and personal growth.

CHAPTER 17

THE CONNECTION BETWEEN ADDICTION AND PSYCHOTIC ILLNESS

Psychotic illness and addiction share a complex, intertwined relationship that has long intrigued and challenged mental health professionals, researchers, and those affected by these conditions. The intersection of these two phenomena is multifaceted and bidirectional, with each condition often exacerbating the other, influenced by biological, psychological, and social factors. Understanding this connection is crucial for prevention, early intervention, and effective treatment. This chapter explores why addiction and psychotic illness often co-occur, the mechanisms that facilitate this connection, and the approaches that can help manage and treat both conditions.

The connection between psychotic illness and addiction

Substance use, particularly drugs like cannabis, amphetamines, and cocaine, can trigger or worsen psychotic symptoms, while individuals with psychotic disorders may turn to substances as a form of self-medication to cope with their distressing symptoms. The underlying mechanisms linking addiction and psychosis often involve neurobiological factors, such as dopamine dysregulation, which is implicated in both conditions. Genetic predispositions, environmental stressors, and the interplay of psychological factors also contribute to the co-occurrence of addiction and psychotic illnesses, complicating both diagnosis and treatment. Addressing these dual diagnoses requires integrated care that targets both conditions simultaneously for more effective outcomes.

Understanding psychosis

Psychosis is a condition characterised by a disconnection from reality that can be a symptom/result of a variety of conditions. People experiencing psychosis may have hallucinations (seeing or hearing things that are not there) and delusions (firmly held false beliefs). Psychotic episodes often disrupt an individual's thinking, emotions, and behaviour, affecting their ability to function normally in daily life. Schizophrenia (see Chapter 18) and bipolar disorder (see Chapter 19) are among the most common psychotic illnesses; however, psychosis can also be linked to severe depression, trauma, or neurological conditions.

The role of substance abuse in psychosis

One of the strongest connections between addiction and psychosis lies in the effects that certain substances can have on the brain. Substances like cannabis, amphetamines, cocaine, and hallucinogens can trigger psychotic symptoms in some individuals. The relationship can be bidirectional – substance abuse may trigger or exacerbate psychosis, and people with psychotic disorders may use substances to cope with their symptoms, thereby developing addiction.

1. **Cannabis and psychosis:** Cannabis, one of the most

commonly used addictive substances, has been linked to an increased risk of psychotic disorders, especially among those who begin using it during adolescence or who have a family history of mental illness. The active ingredient in cannabis, tetrahydrocannabinol (THC), can alter brain chemistry, sometimes resulting in hallucinations, paranoia, and delusional thinking. Repeated use can increase the likelihood of a psychotic disorder manifesting, particularly in those with a genetic predisposition.

2. **Stimulants:** Stimulant drugs like amphetamines and cocaine can also induce psychotic symptoms. These substances increase dopamine levels in the brain, leading to heightened energy, euphoria, and sometimes, aggressive or paranoid behaviour. Chronic use can result in stimulant-induced psychosis, which may present as hallucinations, delusions, and confusion. In some cases, psychotic episodes persist even after the substance has left the system, suggesting a lasting impact on brain function.

Why addiction and psychosis co-occur

Addiction and psychotic illness are often linked through a combination of genetic, neurobiological, and environmental factors:

1. **Genetic vulnerability:** Research indicates that some individuals have a genetic predisposition to both addiction and psychosis. Genes involved in dopamine regulation, for instance, may increase vulnerability to both conditions. The overlap suggests that addiction and psychosis may not only be connected but may also share common roots, making those with one condition at higher risk of developing the other.

2. **Self-medication and coping strategies:** For many

individuals with psychotic illnesses, substances become a coping mechanism. The experience of hallucinations or delusions can be deeply distressing, leading people to seek relief through alcohol, cannabis, or other drugs. This self-medication can provide temporary escape or relief from negative symptoms such as anxiety, depression, and social withdrawal; however, it also increases the risk of addiction.

3. **Neurobiological mechanisms:** Dopamine dysregulation is central to both addiction and psychotic illnesses. In psychosis, particularly in schizophrenia, abnormal dopamine activity is associated with hallucinations and delusions. Similarly, addictive substances like stimulants affect dopamine pathways, reinforcing drug-seeking behaviour. The overlap in these neurobiological mechanisms helps explain why individuals with one condition are at higher risk of developing the other.

The impact of co-occurring addiction and psychosis

When addiction and psychotic illness co-occur, the effects on the individual are profound. Both conditions may exacerbate each other, leading to a vicious cycle of worsening symptoms and increased drug use. This dual diagnosis, also known as 'co-morbidity' or 'dual disorder,' presents unique challenges:

1. **Increased severity of symptoms:** Substance use often worsens the symptoms of psychosis, making them more frequent or severe. Individuals may experience more intense hallucinations, paranoia, and confusion, increasing their risk of harm to themselves or others.

2. **Complicated treatment process:** Treating individuals with both conditions is more challenging than treating either

condition alone. Medications for psychosis may not work as effectively if the individual is using drugs, and withdrawal symptoms can sometimes mimic or intensify psychotic symptoms.

3. **Social and functional impairment:** Co-occurring addiction and psychosis often lead to greater social isolation, unemployment, homelessness, and difficulty maintaining relationships. The stigma associated with both addiction and mental illness compounds these challenges, making it harder for individuals to seek and receive appropriate care.

Prevention and early intervention

Given the intricate relationship between addiction and psychosis, prevention and early intervention are vital. Strategies include:

1. **Educating at-risk populations:** Adolescents, individuals with a family history of mental illness, and people living in high-stress environments would benefit from being educated about the risks associated with substance use. Highlighting the connection between cannabis use and psychosis, for instance, can dissuade vulnerable individuals from experimenting with drugs.

2. **Screening and monitoring:** Early screening for substance use in individuals who show signs of psychosis - or vice versa - can allow for prompt intervention. Mental health services and substance use programmes should work together to create a unified approach to monitoring and supporting high-risk individuals.

3. **Integrated treatment models:** Combining mental health and addiction services is essential for early intervention

and effective treatment. Integrated models that address both conditions simultaneously, using a combination of medication, cognitive behavioural therapy (CBT), and psychosocial support, have shown greater success in managing co-morbidity than treating each condition separately.

Treatment approaches

Treating individuals with co-occurring addiction and psychosis requires a comprehensive, multidisciplinary approach. Key strategies include:

1. **Medications:** Antipsychotic medications are often used to manage psychotic symptoms. However, careful consideration is needed to avoid interactions with substances that the person may be using. In cases of stimulant-induced psychosis, cessation of drug use may resolve symptoms, although ongoing support is necessary to prevent relapse.

2. **Psychotherapy:** CBT is particularly effective for addressing both psychosis and addiction. It helps individuals recognise triggers, develop healthier coping mechanisms, and challenge distorted thinking patterns. Motivational interviewing (MI) is another valuable technique, encouraging individuals to find intrinsic motivation to reduce substance use.

3. **Rehabilitation and social support:** People with dual diagnoses benefit from rehabilitation programmes that include not only medical and psychological care but also social support services. These programmes can help individuals rebuild their lives, find stable housing, and engage in meaningful activities, reducing the risk of relapse.

4. **Harm reduction approaches:** For individuals who may

not be ready to quit substance use entirely, harm reduction strategies can be implemented. This includes supervised consumption services, needle exchanges, and education on safer substance use, minimising the immediate risks while building trust and encouraging treatment engagement.

When to seek help

Recognising the early signs of a worsening psychotic illness is crucial for ensuring timely intervention and preventing further harm. Psychosis can impair an individual's ability to function and can lead to significant distress for both the person affected and their loved ones. If left unaddressed, psychotic symptoms can escalate, so it is important to seek professional help when the following signs arise:

1. **Increasing difficulty in distinguishing reality from hallucinations or delusions:** When an individual finds it increasingly difficult to differentiate between what is real and what is a hallucination or delusion, it may indicate the progression of psychosis. This confusion can impair judgement and decision-making, making intervention essential.

2. **Severe disruption of daily life:** If psychotic symptoms are interfering with an individual's ability to perform daily activities, such as going to work, maintaining personal hygiene, or handling basic tasks, it's important to seek help. This includes instances where the person is unable to care for themselves due to the severity of their symptoms.

3. **Escalating paranoia, aggression, or suicidal thoughts:** A significant increase in paranoid thoughts, aggressive behaviour, or verbal and physical outbursts can be warning signs that the psychosis is worsening. Suicidal thinking or attempts require immediate attention and intervention to

ensure the person's safety.

4. **Social withdrawal and loss of interest in activities:** A noticeable and sudden withdrawal from social interactions, a decline in maintaining relationships, or a complete loss of interest in previously enjoyed activities may suggest an intensification of psychotic symptoms. This social isolation can worsen the individual's condition and further hinder recovery efforts.

Seeking help as soon as these signs are noticed can significantly improve the outcomes for individuals experiencing psychotic illness. Professional care can provide crucial support and prevent further deterioration of mental and emotional wellbeing.

Conclusion

The relationship between addiction and psychotic illness is intricate and frequently misinterpreted. The interplay of genetic predispositions, neurobiological factors, and environmental influences highlights the importance of comprehensive and integrated treatment strategies. By emphasising prevention, early intervention, and personalised, supportive care, mental health services can better tackle the simultaneous occurrence of these disorders, leading to improved outcomes for those impacted.

CHAPTER 18

THE CONNECTION BETWEEN ADDICTION AND SCHIZOPHRENIA

As we saw in the previous chapter, schizophrenia is one of a number of conditions associated with psychosis, and there is a strong connection between psychosis and addiction. Schizophrenia specifically, which involves both psychosis and 'negative symptoms' (see below), and addiction frequently overlap, creating a complicated and deeply interconnected reality for those affected by both. This chapter delves into the relationship between these two conditions, examining the reasons behind this dual diagnosis, the factors that increase its likelihood, and the ways in which individuals can find support. It also highlights effective interventions and strategies for managing the combined challenges of schizophrenia and addiction.

The connection between schizophrenia and addiction

The connection between addiction and schizophrenia is complex and often problematic, with individuals diagnosed with schizophrenia being at a significantly higher risk of developing substance use disorders. This dual diagnosis is believed to arise from several factors, including a tendency for people with schizophrenia to self-medicate with drugs or alcohol to alleviate symptoms such as anxiety, hallucinations, or social isolation. Additionally, shared genetic and neurobiological factors, particularly involving the brain's dopamine system, may contribute to both conditions. The presence of addiction can complicate the treatment of schizophrenia, exacerbating symptoms and impairing recovery, which makes an integrated approach to diagnosis and treatment essential for improving outcomes.

Understanding the connection between addiction and schizophrenia

A dual diagnosis, also known as a co-occurring disorder or 'co-morbidity,' refers to the simultaneous presence of a mental health disorder and a substance use disorder. In the case of schizophrenia and addiction, this connection is particularly profound. Research indicates that people with schizophrenia are significantly more likely to develop substance use disorders than the general population. Studies suggest that between 40 and 50% of individuals with schizophrenia have a history of substance abuse, compared with 8% of the general population.

The question remains: why is there such a strong connection between these two conditions? Several factors contribute, including the attempt to self-medicate, genetic predisposition, environmental triggers, and neurological abnormalities.

How it happens

The relationship between addiction and schizophrenia is multifaceted. Some of the key factors include:

1. **Self-medication hypothesis:** Many individuals with schizophrenia turn to drugs and alcohol as a means to cope with distressing symptoms such as hallucinations, delusions,

or negative emotions like anxiety and depression. This self-medication hypothesis suggests that people use substances to temporarily alleviate their suffering, despite the long-term negative consequences. For example, cannabis is often used by individuals with schizophrenia in an attempt to relax or feel less anxious; however, it can also worsen psychotic symptoms.

2. **Genetic vulnerability:** There is evidence to suggest that genetic factors play a significant role in both schizophrenia and addiction. Certain genes associated with dopamine dysregulation may predispose individuals to both conditions. Dopamine, a neurotransmitter linked to pleasure and reward, is a crucial element in addiction, and it also plays a central role in the development of schizophrenia. This shared genetic vulnerability means that individuals who are genetically predisposed to schizophrenia may also be at higher risk of developing addiction.

3. **Neurological and neurochemical changes:** Schizophrenia and addiction both affect the brain's reward system, specifically the dopaminergic pathways. Substance use can alter these pathways, leading to changes in how the brain responds to stimuli, making individuals more susceptible to addiction. Moreover, chronic substance use can exacerbate or even trigger psychotic symptoms, creating a vicious cycle where addiction worsens schizophrenia and vice versa.

4. **Environmental and social factors:** Environmental factors, such as stress, trauma, and social isolation, are known to increase the risk of both schizophrenia and substance use disorders. Individuals with schizophrenia often experience significant social and occupational difficulties, leading to isolation, marginalisation, and a lack of social support. In

this context, drugs or alcohol may become an accessible means of escape or comfort.

The impact of co-occurring schizophrenia and addiction

The combination of schizophrenia and addiction can have severe consequences for the individual, complicating both diagnosis and treatment. People with dual diagnoses are more likely to experience:

1. **Worsened symptomatology:** Substance use can worsen the symptoms of schizophrenia, leading to more frequent and severe psychotic episodes. It can also make it more difficult for healthcare providers to distinguish between primary symptoms of schizophrenia and those induced by drugs, delaying appropriate treatment.

2. **Reduced treatment adherence:** Addiction often interferes with the individual's ability to adhere to prescribed medications for schizophrenia. For instance, someone using substances like cannabis or stimulants may neglect their antipsychotic medications, resulting in worsening symptoms and an increased likelihood of relapse.

3. **Increased risk of suicide and violence:** The risk of suicide is significantly higher among individuals with co-occurring disorders. The interplay of schizophrenia symptoms, such as paranoia or delusions, with the disinhibiting effects of drugs or alcohol can lead to self-harm or violence towards others. Without appropriate intervention, the combination of these factors can become life-threatening.

Addressing the dual diagnosis

Given the complexity of managing both schizophrenia and addiction, an integrated treatment approach is essential. Treating each disorder in isolation is often ineffective; therefore, both conditions must be addressed simultaneously. Here's how:

1. **Comprehensive assessment and diagnosis:** An accurate diagnosis is the first step in treatment. This requires careful assessment by a multidisciplinary team, including psychiatrists, addiction specialists, and therapists, to distinguish between primary symptoms of schizophrenia and those resulting from substance use. Understanding the individual's pattern of substance use is crucial for developing a personalised treatment plan.

2. **Integrated dual diagnosis treatment:** Treatment for co-occurring disorders should integrate psychiatric care with addiction treatment. This may involve a combination of medication management, psychosocial support, and behavioural therapies. For schizophrenia, antipsychotic medications are typically prescribed to stabilise psychotic symptoms. However, the presence of addiction may necessitate additional interventions, such as detoxification or medications to manage cravings and withdrawal symptoms.

3. **Psychosocial interventions:** Psychosocial interventions, such as cognitive behavioural therapy (CBT) and motivational interviewing, are effective in addressing the behavioural aspects of addiction while helping individuals develop coping strategies for managing schizophrenia. CBT, for instance, can help patients identify and change patterns of thought that contribute to both substance use and psychotic episodes.

4. **Harm reduction and relapse prevention:** In cases where complete abstinence from substances may not be immediately achievable, harm reduction strategies can be implemented. These may include providing safer alternatives, reducing risky behaviours, or minimising the harm associated with continued substance use. Simultaneously, relapse prevention programmes are vital to equip individuals with tools and strategies to manage stressors and cravings that may trigger substance use.

5. **Social support and rehabilitation:** Social isolation is a significant risk factor for both schizophrenia and addiction. Thus, fostering supportive relationships and rebuilding social connections are both essential. Rehabilitation services, such as supported housing and vocational training, can help individuals regain independence and improve their quality of life, reducing the risk of relapse.

When to seek help

Understanding when to seek help for schizophrenia is essential for managing symptoms and improving long-term outcomes. Recognising early signs and reaching out for support can prevent the escalation of symptoms and help individuals lead a better quality of life. Below are key moments when it is crucial to seek professional help for schizophrenia:

1. **Early intervention:** The earlier the intervention, the better the long-term prognosis. If symptoms of schizophrenia, such as hallucinations, delusions, or confusion, begin to interfere with daily functioning, it is important to seek professional help immediately. Early treatment can help prevent the worsening of symptoms and reduce the risk of a more severe episode.

2. **When symptoms worsen:** If an individual's symptoms start to escalate - such as increased paranoia, disorganised thinking, or withdrawal from reality - it is crucial to seek help right away. Delays in treatment can lead to greater difficulty in managing symptoms and may result in hospitalisation.

3. **Difficulty with medication adherence:** If a person with schizophrenia struggles to maintain their medication regimen, it may signal that professional support is needed. Non-adherence to medication can lead to relapse or worsening of symptoms. Mental health professionals can provide guidance, alternatives, and strategies to improve adherence.

4. **Social withdrawal or isolation:** When an individual begins to withdraw from family, friends, or everyday activities, it is important to address the issue promptly. Isolation can worsen symptoms of schizophrenia and increase the risk of depression and other complications. Seeking help early can provide access to social support networks and therapy.

5. **Crisis situations or suicidal thoughts:** If the individual expresses thoughts of harming themselves or others, immediate intervention is crucial. Schizophrenia can sometimes lead to severe distress, and timely professional help, such as through a crisis team or hospitalisation, can prevent harm and stabilise the individual.

Seeking help at the right time is crucial for individuals with schizophrenia to ensure proper treatment and improve their quality of life. Early intervention, recognising worsening symptoms, and addressing challenges such as medication adherence or isolation can make a significant difference in managing the condition. Always seek professional guidance when in doubt, as timely support can lead to more effective management of schizophrenia.

Conclusion

In managing co-occurring schizophrenia and addiction, a holistic approach that encompasses medication, therapy, social support, and lifestyle changes is essential. It is not just about treating symptoms; it's about fostering resilience, encouraging social reintegration, and building a sustainable pathway to recovery.

Living with a dual diagnosis presents immense challenges; however, with the right interventions and support, individuals can manage both conditions, improve their quality of life, and reclaim their independence. A proactive, empathetic approach involving healthcare providers, families, and the wider community is essential to ensure that those affected by the intersection of schizophrenia and addiction receive the care they need to thrive.

CHAPTER 19

THE CONNECTION BETWEEN ADDICTION AND BIPOLAR DISORDER

Bipolar disorder and addiction frequently occur together, and the relationship between them is intricate and multi-dimensional, as we have seen in psychosis (Chapter 17) and schizophrenia (Chapter 18). Understanding why these conditions are so often linked is crucial for anyone dealing with either of these challenges. This chapter explores the nature of this connection, why it happens, how it manifests, and what steps can be taken to address it effectively.

The connection between bipolar disorder and addiction

As we have seen with other mental health conditions, people with bipolar disorder may turn to substances as a way to self-medicate, either to manage the extreme mood swings of mania or to cope with the despair of depressive episodes. This self-medication often exacerbates the symptoms of both disorders, creating a vicious cycle that is difficult to break. The underlying causes of this connection include genetic, neurobiological, and psychological factors that contribute to impulsivity, risk-taking behaviours, and a heightened vulnerability to addiction. As a result, effective treatment requires an integrated approach that addresses both the mood disorder and the substance use issue simultaneously.

Understanding bipolar disorder and addiction

Bipolar disorder is a mental health condition characterised by extreme mood swings, including manic or hypomanic episodes (periods of elevated mood, energy, and activity levels) and depressive episodes (periods of intense sadness, hopelessness, or lethargy). Addiction, or substance use disorder, involves the compulsive use of substances, like alcohol, drugs, or behaviours, like gambling, despite harmful consequences. Both conditions significantly impact an individual's behaviour, emotions, and daily life.

Research suggests that individuals with bipolar disorder are more likely to struggle with addiction. Approximately 50–60% of those with bipolar disorder may experience a substance use disorder at some point in their lives. This co-morbidity presents a severe challenge as it often worsens the symptoms of both conditions, making treatment more complex.

How it happens

The link between addiction and bipolar disorder can be attributed to several factors, including genetic, biological, psychological, and social influences:

1. **Self-medication hypothesis:** As we have seen with other mental health problems, many individuals with bipolar disorder use substances as a means of self-medication. For those experiencing intense emotional highs or debilitating lows, alcohol or drugs might seem like a useful way to regulate their mood. For instance, during depressive episodes, substances like alcohol or opioids may be used to

numb emotional pain, while during manic episodes, stimulants or other drugs might be sought to amplify feelings of euphoria.

2. **Neurobiological factors:** Both addiction and bipolar disorder involve dysfunctions in brain chemistry, particularly in the areas related to reward processing, mood regulation, and impulse control. Neurotransmitters like dopamine and serotonin play critical roles in mood stability and are also central to the brain's response to addictive substances. This overlap means that individuals with bipolar disorder are biologically more susceptible to addiction, as their brain's reward systems might seek external stimuli (substances) to achieve a sense of balance or pleasure.

3. **Genetic predisposition:** Genetic studies suggest that the same genes that increase the risk of developing bipolar disorder may also predispose individuals to addiction. If someone has a family history of either condition, they are more likely to develop both, indicating that the two share common genetic factors.

4. **Impulse control issues:** During manic or hypomanic phases, individuals with bipolar disorder often experience heightened impulsivity, risk-taking behaviours, and reduced inhibitions. These states can lead to experimentation with drugs or alcohol as the individual seeks new experiences or heightened sensations. In such moments, the impulsivity associated with mania can fuel substance abuse, which may become a chronic habit even after the manic episode ends.

5. **Psychosocial influences:** Social and environmental factors also play a role. Individuals with bipolar disorder may

struggle with maintaining relationships, holding down jobs, or staying engaged with their communities due to the instability caused by mood swings. Substance use can become a coping mechanism for managing these difficulties or a way to fit into social groups that also engage in substance use.

How the connection manifests

When addiction and bipolar disorder co-occur, they often create a vicious cycle. Substance abuse can worsen the mood instability seen in bipolar disorder, triggering more frequent or severe manic and depressive episodes. At the same time, untreated bipolar symptoms can lead to increased substance use as the person tries to manage or escape their mood states. For example:

1. **During manic episodes:** Individuals may use stimulants, alcohol, or other substances to intensify their elevated mood or to prolong the high-energy state. This can lead to dangerous behaviour, increased risk-taking, and even physical harm.

2. **During depressive episodes:** The craving for relief can drive individuals to use depressants, like alcohol or sedatives, to escape the overwhelming sadness or emptiness. However, this temporary relief often leads to dependence and a worsening of depressive symptoms.

This cycle not only complicates diagnosis; it also makes treatment more challenging, as healthcare professionals need to address both conditions simultaneously. When addiction is not managed, it often leads to non-compliance with bipolar medication, and when bipolar disorder is untreated, it heightens the risk of relapse into substance use.

Chapter 19

What can be done for treatment and support

The coexistence of addiction and bipolar disorder requires a comprehensive, integrated approach. Here's how to manage and treat both conditions effectively:

1. **Seek integrated treatment:** The most effective way to manage co-occurring bipolar disorder and addiction is through integrated treatment programmes that address both conditions simultaneously. This includes a combination of medication, therapy, and support that focuses on stabilising mood and managing substance use.
    - **Medication:** Mood stabilisers like lithium, anticonvulsants, or antipsychotics, are often used to control bipolar symptoms, while other medications may be prescribed to help reduce cravings or withdrawal symptoms from substances. Close monitoring is essential, as some medications used for addiction can interact negatively with bipolar treatments.
    - **Psychotherapy:** Cognitive behavioural therapy (CBT) and dialectical behaviour therapy (DBT) are particularly effective for individuals with co-occurring disorders. CBT helps individuals recognise and change harmful patterns of thought and behaviour, while DBT focuses on emotional regulation and coping strategies, which are crucial for managing both mood swings and addiction triggers.

2. **Build a support network:** Building a support network is critical. Family members, friends, and support groups can offer the emotional stability and encouragement needed during recovery. Connecting with others who understand bipolar disorder and addiction can reduce feelings of isolation and provide practical advice and support.

3. **Maintain a routine and healthy lifestyle:** Structure and routine are important for individuals managing both conditions. Establishing a regular sleep schedule, maintaining a balanced diet, and engaging in physical activity can stabilise mood and reduce the desire for substances. Avoiding triggers, such as environments or social circles that encourage substance use, is also key.

4. **Relapse prevention strategies:** Relapse is common in both addiction (see Chapter 10) and bipolar disorder, so developing prevention strategies is crucial. This includes learning to identify warning signs of mood episodes or cravings, managing stress through healthy outlets like mindfulness or exercise, and having an emergency plan in place if symptoms worsen.

5. **Consistent monitoring and follow-up:** Regular follow-up appointments with healthcare providers ensure that treatment remains effective and adjustments can be made as needed. Monitoring not only helps maintain mood stability; it also ensures any signs of relapse are caught early and managed promptly.

When to seek help

Recognising the signs of bipolar disorder and seeking help early are crucial for managing the condition effectively. Bipolar disorder can have a significant impact on daily life and relationships, so timely intervention is essential to prevent the condition from escalating. If symptoms are left untreated, they can lead to severe mood episodes and complications such as substance abuse or other co-occurring disorders. Here are key moments when professional help should be sought:

1. **Severe mood swings or emotional instability:** If you or someone you know is experiencing dramatic shifts in mood, from intense feelings of euphoria or irritability during manic episodes to deep sadness or hopelessness during depressive episodes, it's important to seek professional help. These mood changes can disrupt personal, social, and work life, and may indicate the need for a mood stabiliser or other treatment options.

2. **Impulsivity and risk-taking behaviours:** During manic episodes, individuals with bipolar disorder may engage in reckless behaviours, such as excessive spending, promiscuity, or substance abuse. If these behaviours become more frequent or intense, seeking help is crucial to prevent harm and ensure that the person gets the support they need to manage their impulses.

3. **Difficulty maintaining daily functioning:** Bipolar disorder can interfere with daily tasks, such as holding down a job, maintaining relationships, or managing basic self-care. If the symptoms of bipolar disorder are making it difficult to function in everyday life, it is essential to consult a mental health professional for an evaluation and appropriate intervention.

4. **Increased substance use or self-medication:** If someone with bipolar disorder starts using alcohol, drugs, or other substances more frequently in an attempt to manage their mood, this may indicate a developing addiction. Substance use can worsen the symptoms of bipolar disorder, so it's important to seek professional help at the first signs of this behaviour.

5. **Thoughts of self-harm or suicide:** In both manic and

depressive episodes, individuals with bipolar disorder may experience thoughts of self-harm or suicide. If these thoughts arise, immediate help should be sought from a mental health professional or helpline. Early intervention can provide critical support and reduce the risk of self-harm or injury.

6. **Family history of bipolar disorder or addiction:** If there is a family history of bipolar disorder or substance use disorders, the individual may be at higher risk. Early awareness of symptoms can lead to earlier diagnosis and more effective management, preventing the condition from worsening.

For those already diagnosed with bipolar disorder, it is important to look out for any signs of substance abuse. Similarly, individuals with a history of addiction should be aware of any mood changes that might suggest the onset of bipolar disorder, as early diagnosis and treatment significantly improve outcomes.

Conclusion

The relationship between addiction and bipolar disorder is intricate, yet grasping this connection is crucial for effective management. By examining the neurobiological, psychological, and social factors that intertwine these conditions, individuals and their families can collaborate with healthcare professionals to create comprehensive and integrated treatment plans. Prioritising early intervention, cultivating a robust support network, and maintaining a dedicated approach to managing both disorders can pave the way for a healthier, more stable life.

CHAPTER 20

THE CONNECTION BETWEEN ADDICTION AND DEPRESSION

Depression and addiction often go hand in hand, forming a complex, self-sustaining pattern that makes both conditions more difficult to manage. Understanding the relationship between them is crucial for effective treatment and prevention. This chapter looks at the factors that link addiction and depression, how this bond develops, and strategies for breaking the cycle. We also discuss the importance of seeking help and treating both conditions together.

The connection between depression and addiction

Depression can lead individuals to use substances or engage in addictive behaviours as a way to cope with feelings of sadness, hopelessness, or emotional pain. While substances may provide temporary relief, they can exacerbate depressive symptoms over time, creating a vicious cycle where addiction deepens depression, and depression fuels further addiction. This interplay is driven by both psychological factors, such as negative thought patterns, and biological factors, including changes in brain chemistry. As we have seen with other mental health issues in previous chapters, addressing both conditions simultaneously is crucial for effective treatment and recovery.

How addiction and depression are interlinked

Addiction and depression are deeply interconnected, often occurring together in what is known as a 'dual diagnosis' or 'co-morbidity'. Studies suggest that people who suffer from depression are more likely to develop addictions, while those with addictions have an increased risk of becoming depressed. This relationship is complex and influenced by a range of biological, psychological, and social factors:

1. **Self-medication and coping:** Depression can leave individuals feeling hopeless, isolated, and emotionally overwhelmed. In an attempt to escape or manage these feelings, many people turn to substances like alcohol or drugs, or behaviours like gambling or excessive gaming. These substances or behaviours provide temporary relief, numbing the emotional pain associated with depression. However, they ultimately worsen the condition, leading to a cycle where more of the substance or behaviour is needed to achieve the same effect.

2. **Biological overlap:** Addiction and depression share some of the same pathways in the brain, particularly those involving neurotransmitters like serotonin and dopamine. Low levels of serotonin are often linked to depression, while dopamine plays a central role in the brain's reward system. Substances such as alcohol, opiates, and stimulants can temporarily increase dopamine levels, providing a short-term sense of euphoria or relief. However, with repeated use, these substances can deplete the brain's natural dopamine reserves, deepening depression and increasing the person's reliance on the substance.

3. **Genetic factors:** Genetics play a significant role in predisposing individuals to both addiction and depression. Those with a family history of either condition are at greater risk. Certain genetic traits may lead to lower levels of neurotransmitters or increased vulnerability to stress, which in turn increases the likelihood of both addiction and depression.

4. **Trauma and environmental stressors:** Trauma, particularly in early life, is a major risk factor for both conditions. Individuals who have experienced abuse, neglect, or other significant traumas may turn to substances as a way of managing their emotions. In addition, ongoing environmental stressors - such as financial difficulties (see Chapter 24), relationship breakdowns (see Chapter 27), or social isolation - can also contribute to the development of depression and the subsequent use of substances as a coping mechanism.

How the cycle of addiction and depression develops

The link between addiction and depression can lead to a harmful cycle, where each condition exacerbates the other. This cycle often follows these stages:

1. **Seeking relief through substances or behaviours:** A person suffering from depression may begin using substances or engaging in addictive behaviours to alleviate feelings of sadness, anxiety, or emptiness. Initially, these may provide temporary relief, offering a sense of escape or euphoria.

2. **Rebound depression and worsening symptoms:** The effects of substances or behaviours are short-lived. When they wear off, the individual is often left feeling worse than

before. Withdrawal symptoms, physical side effects, and the realisation of reliance on these substances can intensify depressive symptoms, reinforcing the need for further use.

3. **Increased dependence and escalation:** Over time, the individual may find that they need higher doses or more frequent engagement with the addictive behaviour to achieve the same effect. This leads to increased dependence, and as the addiction deepens, the negative consequences accumulate - further isolation, health issues, and damage to relationships - all of which feed into, and amplify, the cycle of depression.

How this connection happens

The connection between addiction and depression is not coincidental; it is often a direct result of the interplay between psychological vulnerabilities, biological predispositions, and environmental influences:

1. **Psychological factors:** Depression can distort a person's thinking, leading them to believe that substances or behaviours are the only way to feel relief or pleasure. These cognitive distortions can make people more susceptible to addiction as they seek to escape their reality.

2. **Biological factors:** Changes in brain chemistry caused by both conditions reinforce each other. For example, chronic use of substances can alter brain function, making it more challenging to experience pleasure naturally, thereby deepening depression.

3. **Social and environmental factors:** Lack of support, social isolation, or stressful life events can trigger depression. For

some, the social environments associated with substance use may offer a sense of belonging, further entrenching the cycle.

What can be done to break the cycle

Addressing the connection between addiction and depression requires a comprehensive, integrated approach. Here are the key steps to break the cycle and achieve recovery:

1. **Professional intervention:** Seeking help from a qualified professional is critical. Therapists, psychologists, and psychiatrists who specialise in co-occurring disorders can provide integrated treatment, addressing both addiction and depression simultaneously. Cognitive behavioural therapy (CBT) and other evidence-based therapies like dialectical behaviour therapy (DBT) are effective in helping individuals manage negative thoughts and develop healthy coping strategies.

2. **Medication:** In some cases, medication may be necessary to stabilise mood and reduce withdrawal symptoms. Antidepressants, when prescribed appropriately, can help balance neurotransmitters like serotonin and dopamine, making it easier to manage depressive symptoms without turning to addictive substances. Medication-assisted treatment (MAT) may also be used for those with substance dependencies, such as opioids or alcohol, to reduce cravings and support recovery.

3. **Developing healthy coping mechanisms:** Learning and practising healthy coping strategies is essential for managing both depression and addiction. Techniques such as mindfulness, relaxation exercises, and physical activities can improve mood and reduce reliance on addictive

behaviours. Engaging in creative pursuits or finding hobbies that provide enjoyment and fulfilment can also serve as positive outlets.

4. **Building a support network:** Addiction and depression often thrive in isolation. Reaching out to trusted friends, family, or support groups can create a network of support that is vital for recovery. Engaging in group therapy or joining organisations such as Alcoholics Anonymous (AA) or Narcotics Anonymous (NA) can provide a sense of community and accountability, while also sharing experiences with others facing similar challenges.

5. **Addressing underlying trauma:** For many, the root of their addiction and depression lies in unresolved trauma. Trauma-informed therapies, such as eye movement desensitisation and reprocessing (EMDR) or trauma-focused CBT, can be effective in processing and healing these past wounds, thereby reducing the reliance on substances or addictive behaviours as a coping mechanism.

6. **Establishing a healthy routine:** Physical activity, good nutrition, and adequate sleep (see Chapter 15) are essential components of recovery. Regular exercise has been shown to boost mood and improve overall wellbeing. Establishing a balanced routine can also provide structure and stability, which is particularly important when managing both addiction and depression.

When to seek help

Depression can be overwhelming, and recognising when professional help is needed is crucial to prevent the condition from worsening. While everyone experiences low moods from time to time, persistent or severe symptoms may signal the need for intervention. The sooner you seek help, the more effectively you can address the condition and begin the path to recovery.

1. **Persistent feelings of hopelessness, sadness, or worthlessness:** If feelings of sadness, despair, or worthlessness persist for weeks or longer, it may be a sign of clinical depression. These emotions can cloud your ability to function in daily life and make it difficult to see a way forward.

2. **Increasing reliance on substances or behaviours to cope:** Turning to substances or engaging in addictive behaviours to numb or manage emotional pain are common responses to depression. If either becomes a habitual coping mechanism, it can worsen both the depression and any accompanying addiction.

3. **Withdrawal from social activities, work, or relationships:** Depression often leads to a loss of interest in activities that were once enjoyable or fulfilling. If you find yourself isolating from family, friends, or colleagues, this could be a sign that depression is taking a significant toll on your life.

4. **Thoughts of self-harm or suicide:** If you or someone you know is experiencing thoughts of self-harm or suicide, it is crucial to seek immediate professional help. These thoughts are serious and require urgent attention to ensure safety and begin appropriate treatment.

5. **Physical symptoms like changes in sleep, appetite, or weight:** Depression often manifests in physical ways, including disruptions to sleep patterns, changes in appetite, and unexplained weight loss or gain. These physical signs can be a direct result of depression and may require medical attention.

Early intervention can make a significant difference in breaking the cycle of depression. The sooner you seek help, the better the chances of preventing the condition from becoming entrenched and improving overall wellbeing.

Conclusion

The connection between addiction and depression is powerful; however, it is not unbreakable. By understanding how these conditions reinforce each other and seeking comprehensive, integrated treatment, individuals can begin the journey towards recovery. While it requires commitment, perseverance, and support, breaking free from this cycle opens up the possibility of a healthier, more fulfilling life. Recognising the signs, taking action early, and building a strong support system are key steps in overcoming the grip of addiction and depression.

CHAPTER 21

THE CONNECTION BETWEEN ADDICTION AND ANXIETY

Addiction and anxiety are deeply intertwined, with each one often fuelling and amplifying the other. The relationship between these two conditions can be complex and multi-faceted, creating a vicious cycle that traps individuals in patterns of substance misuse and mental health struggles. As with other mental health problems (see Chapters 16 to 19), understanding the connection between addiction and anxiety is crucial for those looking to break free from these destructive cycles and regain control over their lives.

The connection between anxiety and addiction

Many individuals turn to substances or addictive behaviours as a way to self-medicate, seeking relief from the overwhelming stress and fear caused by anxiety. While substances may provide temporary calm or euphoria, they ultimately worsen anxiety over time, creating a cycle of dependence. As tolerance builds, more of the substance is needed to achieve the same effect, while withdrawal can intensify feelings of anxiety, leading to a reinforcing loop. This interplay highlights the need for integrated treatment that addresses both the anxiety and addiction simultaneously, breaking the cycle and fostering long-term recovery.

How anxiety and addiction are linked

At the most basic level, addiction and anxiety are both conditions that involve disruptions in how the brain manages emotions, stress, and pleasure. They often co-occur because one can exacerbate the symptoms of the other. For many people, addiction is a form of self-medication - a way to alleviate the overwhelming feelings of anxiety. Substances like alcohol, drugs, or even behaviours like gambling or overeating can temporarily dull feelings of fear, worry, or panic.

However, while substances may provide short-term relief, they inevitably worsen anxiety in the long run. The body and mind develop tolerance, meaning more of the substance is required to achieve the same effect. Simultaneously, withdrawal symptoms, including increased anxiety, start to emerge when the substance is absent. This process sets up a dangerous cycle where the individual becomes more dependent on the addictive behaviour or substance to manage their worsening anxiety.

How the connection happens

The brain's response to stress and pleasure is central to understanding how addiction and anxiety become linked. When we experience anxiety, our brain's stress response is activated, releasing hormones like cortisol and adrenaline. These chemicals prepare the body for a 'fight-or-flight' response; however, when anxiety is chronic, the body is perpetually flooded with these hormones, creating a state of ongoing tension and discomfort.

To counteract these feelings, people often turn to substances or addictive behaviours that temporarily increase levels of dopamine, the brain's 'feel-good' chemical. Alcohol, for example, can initially reduce inhibitions and relax the body, while drugs like benzodiazepines (prescribed for anxiety) or opioids flood the brain with dopamine, providing a sense of calm and pleasure. These substances mask the feelings of anxiety; however, they don't address the underlying cause. As tolerance builds, the calming effects wear off more quickly, and the brain's natural ability to regulate stress and pleasure becomes impaired. The individual is then caught in a cycle of needing more of the substance to feel normal, while the absence of it heightens anxiety.

Why is there a connection between anxiety and addiction

There are several reasons why anxiety and addiction are so closely related, with many of the root causes overlapping.

1. **Genetic predisposition:** Genetic makeup plays a significant role in both anxiety disorders and addiction. Studies have shown that individuals with a family history of either condition are more likely to develop the other. Genetic factors influence how our brain chemistry reacts to stress, making some people more vulnerable to both anxiety and substance use disorders.

2. **Environmental stressors:** Traumatic events, chronic stress, and adverse childhood experiences are often shared triggers for both anxiety and addiction. Individuals who have been exposed to prolonged stress or trauma may turn to substances as a way of coping, creating a dependency that can be difficult to break.

3. **Mental health stigma:** In many cultures, including in the UK, there is still a lingering stigma surrounding mental health issues. Individuals who struggle with anxiety may feel embarrassed or ashamed to seek help, pushing them toward substances that seem to offer immediate relief.

Unfortunately, this only deepens their dependence and exacerbates their anxiety.

4. **Cognitive factors:** People with anxiety often have negative thought patterns, such as catastrophising or obsessive worry. These thought patterns can make individuals feel helpless and overwhelmed, leading them to seek escape through substance use. Conversely, the shame and guilt that accompany addiction can fuel more anxious thoughts, perpetuating the cycle.

What to do

Breaking the connection between addiction and anxiety requires addressing both conditions simultaneously. Focusing only on one aspect of the problem may provide temporary relief; however, lasting recovery is unlikely unless both anxiety and addiction are treated in tandem. Here's a roadmap for how to approach this process:

1. **Seek professional help:** The most important step in managing addiction and anxiety is seeking professional support. Cognitive behavioural therapy (CBT) and dialectical behaviour therapy (DBT) among a range of therapeutic approaches have been shown to be effective for both conditions. Working with a counsellor or therapist helps individuals develop healthy coping mechanisms for managing anxiety, without resorting to addictive substances or behaviours.

2. **Address the root cause:** Anxiety often stems from unresolved emotional issues or past trauma. Therapy can provide a safe space to explore these issues, allowing the individual to confront their fears and anxieties in a healthy, constructive way. Identifying triggers and developing strategies to

manage them is crucial in preventing relapse into addictive behaviour.

3. **Consider medication:** For some people, medication may be necessary to help regulate anxiety and prevent relapse into addiction. However, this should be carefully monitored by a medical professional, especially given the risk of dependency on certain anti-anxiety medications. Medications such as antidepressants or non-addictive anti-anxiety medications may provide relief without contributing to the cycle of addiction.

4. **Develop healthy coping strategies:** Learning new ways to manage anxiety without resorting to addictive substances is a key aspect of recovery. Techniques like mindfulness, meditation, and deep breathing can help calm the mind and reduce feelings of panic or worry. Regular physical exercise, which releases endorphins and lowers stress levels, is also beneficial for both mental health and overcoming addiction.

5. **Build a support network:** Having a strong support network can make a world of difference in recovery. Friends, family, and support groups provide accountability and encouragement. They can offer perspective when anxiety feels overwhelming, and they can help individuals stay on track with their recovery goals.

When to seek help

Anxiety can have a significant impact on various aspects of life; recognising the signs that it's time to seek professional help is crucial. Timely intervention can prevent anxiety from becoming more severe and help manage it effectively. Below are specific situations where seeking help is recommended:

1. **Interference with daily life:** If anxiety is preventing you/your loved one from managing everyday tasks, such as going to work, maintaining relationships, or taking care of personal responsibilities, it's time to seek professional support.

2. **Persistent symptoms:** When anxiety symptoms continue for weeks or months and do not seem to improve, professional intervention may be necessary to provide the right treatment and support.

3. **Overwhelming physical symptoms:** If anxiety is causing persistent physical symptoms like headaches, digestive issues, or muscle tension that do not improve, seeking professional help can prevent long-term health consequences.

4. **Reliance on substances for relief:** If you/your loved one begin/s using alcohol, drugs, or other substances to cope with anxiety, it's essential to seek support before this behaviour develops into an addiction.

5. **Frequent panic attacks:** Regular panic attacks, marked by overwhelming fear or physical symptoms like rapid heartbeat, dizziness, or shortness of breath, require immediate professional attention.

6. **Avoidance of everyday activities:** If anxiety leads to avoidance of situations, people, or places that are important to your life, professional support can help you confront and manage these fears.

7. **Strained relationships:** If anxiety is causing difficulties in communication or relationships, therapy can help improve interpersonal skills and reduce the impact of anxiety on social connections.

No matter how long anxiety has been affecting your life, it's never too late to reach out for support. With the right treatment and commitment, managing anxiety becomes possible, and a healthier, more balanced life can be achieved.

My personal experience

Living in a constant state of tension was exhausting. The anxious thoughts often fuelled an urgent need to keep moving forward, pushing me to keep going, even when my body pleaded for rest. I never understood why I was so tired and why I would catch my breath; now I understand that this was a major factor. The constant need for perfection and achievement only heighted my anxiety. Understanding that cycle allowed me to introduce calming practices into my daily life. That shift gave me a renewed sense of control over my wellbeing.

Conclusion

The link between addiction and anxiety is undeniable, with one condition often feeding into the other in a vicious cycle. Understanding this connection is the first step towards breaking free from it. By addressing both anxiety and addiction together, whether through therapy, medication, or lifestyle changes, individuals can begin to regain control over their lives and find healthier, more sustainable ways to manage stress. Recovery is possible, although it requires courage, support, and a willingness to confront both anxiety and addiction head-on.

PART II(B)

THE CONNECTION TO ADDICTION: OUR ENVIRONMENT

To be yourself in a world that is constantly trying to make you something else is the greatest accomplishment.

Ralph Waldo Emerson, philosopher, writer and abolitionist, 1803–1882

CHAPTER 22

THE CONNECTION BETWEEN ADDICTION AND OUR ENVIRONMENT

Addiction is often perceived as an individual problem, a personal struggle to overcome internal cravings, dependencies, or habits. However, this viewpoint overlooks the profound impact that the external world - our environment - has on the development and persistence of addictive behaviours. From the people we interact with, to the socio-economic structures we live within, to the media we consume, the environment plays a pivotal role in shaping our relationship with substances or behaviours that may lead to addiction. In this chapter, we explore how and why this connection between addiction and environment occurs, what drives it, and, crucially, how we can intervene to break the cycle of addiction.

The connection between our environment and addiction

Our environment is a powerful force that profoundly shapes our behaviours, including our susceptibility to addiction. It encompasses not only our physical surroundings but also the social, cultural, and economic conditions that influence our daily lives. The relationships we nurture, the communities we belong to, and even the messages we absorb from media and technology all contribute to the pressures and choices we face. These factors can either foster resilience or create vulnerabilities that increase the risk of addiction. Understanding how our environment shapes these behaviours is essential for addressing the root causes of addiction and creating pathways to healthier lives.

The role of environment in shaping behaviour

To understand the connection between addiction and the environment, we must first recognise that human beings are social creatures. Our behaviours are not developed in isolation; they are moulded by the context in which we live. The environment encompasses physical surroundings, social networks, cultural norms, economic conditions, and even political structures. Each of these factors plays a part in creating a landscape that can either foster resilience or contribute to vulnerability to addiction.

1. **Social environment:** Our relationships with others - family, friends, colleagues, and even the broader community - have a significant impact on our behaviour. A toxic or stressful home environment, social isolation, or peer pressure can increase susceptibility to addictive behaviours. If we are surrounded by people who normalise or engage in substance use, gambling, or other compulsive behaviours, it becomes easier to justify or adopt those habits ourselves.

2. **Cultural and societal norms:** Cultural values can shape what is considered acceptable or normal behaviour. In societies where drinking alcohol or recreational drug use is a common part of social gatherings, individuals may be more likely to engage in these activities. In contrast, cultures that value sobriety or moderation might offer protective factors against addiction. Society's attitudes towards mental health

and addiction (see Chapter 2) also matter. In environments where seeking help is stigmatised, individuals might hide their struggles, preventing early intervention.

3. **Economic and physical environment:** Poverty, unemployment, and limited access to education or healthcare are often strongly linked to addiction. Financial stress, lack of opportunity, and environments where drugs or alcohol are easily accessible can create a fertile ground for addiction to thrive. Deprived neighbourhoods with higher rates of crime, unemployment, and substance availability tend to have higher rates of addiction. Additionally, living in areas where recreational activities are limited may push individuals to seek out substances or behaviours as a form of escapism.

4. **Media and technology:** Modern technology and the media also have a profound influence on addictive behaviour. From advertising that glamourises alcohol and fast food to social media platforms designed to keep users hooked, our digital environment is constantly shaping our habits. The rise of internet-based addictions, such as gambling and gaming, has grown exponentially, largely driven by the fact that these activities are now easily accessible, normalised, and highly engaging.

Why our environment and addiction are so closely linked

The link between environment and addiction is crucial to understanding the factors that contribute to addictive behaviours. Our surroundings play a significant role in shaping our experiences, stress levels, and coping mechanisms.

1. **Stress and coping mechanisms:** One of the key reasons why the environment plays such a central role in addiction is due to its impact on stress levels. Stress (see Chapter 25), whether it stems from financial difficulties, emotional trauma, or social isolation, is a well-known trigger for addictive behaviour. Our environment shapes how much stress we experience and how we are equipped to cope with it. For some, turning to substances or compulsive behaviours offers a way to escape, albeit temporarily, from overwhelming feelings. If the environment consistently induces high levels of stress without offering healthy coping strategies, the risk of addiction increases.

2. **Availability and accessibility:** Another reason the environment contributes to addiction is the availability and accessibility of addictive substances or behaviours. If you live in an area where drugs are readily available, or where gambling shops, fast-food chains, or alcohol outlets are prevalent, there is a greater temptation to engage in those activities. The convenience of access lowers the barriers to entry, increasing the likelihood of use and, over time, addiction.

3. **The influence of social learning:** Addiction can also be understood through the lens of social learning theory, which suggests that individuals learn behaviours by observing others. If addiction is prevalent in one's immediate environment – whether it's family members drinking excessively or friends who gamble regularly – it becomes normalised. These patterns of behaviour are internalised, and individuals may adopt them, consciously or unconsciously.

4. **The normalisation of escapism:** Modern life, with its relentless pace, economic pressures, and digital distractions, has

normalised a culture of escapism. Many environments promote the idea that to relax, cope, or socialise, one must engage with substances like alcohol, drugs, or even technology. This societal norm makes it easier to justify over indulgent or excessive behaviour, which, over time, can spiral into addiction.

What can be done to address the environmental factors

To break the link between addiction and the environment, a multifaceted approach is needed. Individuals, communities, and policymakers all have roles to play in reshaping the environmental conditions that contribute to addiction. Here's what you can do:

1. **Building resilient social networks:** One of the most effective ways to combat addiction is through fostering strong, supportive social environments. Families, friends, and communities can create an atmosphere where individuals feel supported, understood, and connected. Encouraging open communication about mental health and addiction, reducing stigma, and promoting healthy coping mechanisms can all help create environments where addiction struggles are less likely to emerge.

2. **Creating safe physical environments:** Addressing the environmental factors that lead to addiction means improving access to healthy, safe spaces. We can all play a part in encouraging governments and local authorities to invest in deprived areas, increasing access to mental health services, providing education and employment opportunities, and regulating the sale of addictive substances. Additionally, providing safe and engaging alternatives for recreation can give individuals, especially young people, more positive outlets for stress relief.

3. **Shaping healthier media environments:** Again, we can put pressure on governments and organisations to regulate media environments that glamourise or promote addictive behaviours. Stricter advertising regulations, particularly regarding alcohol, gambling, and fast food, can help reduce exposure to these behaviours. Additionally, educational campaigns can be designed to promote awareness of the dangers of addiction and provide resources for seeking help.

4. **Policy and community action:** We must ask our governments and community leaders to take proactive steps to reduce the environmental factors that contribute to addiction. This can include better regulation of substances, limiting the number of alcohol and gambling outlets in a given area, and providing financial assistance or employment support for those in economically vulnerable situations. Communities themselves can initiate localised addiction prevention programmes, offering education, outreach, and intervention efforts.

When to seek help

Understanding when to address the environmental factors that contribute to addiction is crucial for effective prevention. The earlier the intervention, the better the chance of preventing addiction from taking hold.

1. **Early childhood:** Environment plays a crucial role in the development of behaviours in early childhood. Creating supportive, stable, and nurturing environments for children - both at home and in schools - can significantly reduce the risk of future addiction. Early education about healthy coping strategies, emotional intelligence, and the dangers

of addiction can foster resilience.

2. **During periods of high stress:** Moments of crisis or stress, such as unemployment, divorce, or trauma, can trigger the onset of addiction. Intervening during these critical periods by offering support, contacting a health professional, and offering stress management resources can help mitigate the risks.

3. **When environmental cues are present:** If you or someone you know is in an environment where addictive substances or behaviours are prevalent, early intervention is essential. Recognising the impact of these cues and making conscious efforts to remove or minimise exposure to them can prevent addiction from developing.

Early intervention, whether in childhood, during periods of stress, or when facing environmental triggers, can significantly reduce the risk of addiction taking hold. By understanding the importance of a supportive environment and taking proactive steps to create healthier surroundings, we can break the cycle of addiction and foster long-term wellbeing.

Conclusion

The environment we live in is deeply intertwined with the development of addiction. From social pressures to economic conditions to media influence, the external world shapes our internal behaviours in profound ways. By understanding the connection between addiction and our environment, we can take proactive steps to reshape the factors that contribute to addiction, creating healthier, more supportive spaces for individuals to thrive in. Whether at the personal, community, or policy level, we all have a role to play in breaking the cycle of addiction and fostering resilience against its grip.

CHAPTER 23

THE CONNECTION BETWEEN ADDICTION AND CONTROL

Addiction is often described as a loss of control. When individuals become addicted, they struggle to regulate their behaviour, emotions, or thoughts. Whether it's substance use, gambling, or even technology, addiction represents a state where control has been relinquished. Yet, paradoxically, addiction often coexists with another behavioural pattern: being overly controlling. This chapter explores the intricate relationship between addiction and the compulsion to control, how one may fuel the other, and strategies to manage these dynamics.

The connection between control and addiction

On the surface, addiction is often characterised by a loss of control – an inability to regulate behaviours or resist urges. Yet, beneath this lies a complex relationship where the need for control, whether over emotions, circumstances, or others, often serves as a driving force for addictive behaviours. Many individuals turn to addiction as a way to manage or escape the anxiety of feeling powerless, creating a cycle where addiction and control feed into one another. Understanding this connection is essential for breaking free from both the grip of addiction and the unhealthy patterns of excessive control, paving the way for a balanced and sustainable recovery.

Understanding control and the need for certainty

Control, in its simplest form, is the ability to regulate or influence situations, people, or outcomes. It provides a sense of stability and certainty in an unpredictable world. For most of us, a certain level of control is necessary for everyday functioning. It helps us navigate life, make decisions, and feel secure. However, when control becomes excessive, rigid, or obsessive, it often signals deeper emotional struggles.

Individuals who exhibit overly controlling behaviour often do so because of fear – fear of the unknown, fear of failure, or fear of being vulnerable. Controlling their environment or others around them provides a temporary sense of safety. Yet this drive for control can become toxic, especially when it spills over into relationships, personal wellbeing, and even into addictive behaviours.

How addiction and control interconnect

At first glance, it may seem contradictory to suggest that addiction, marked by an apparent lack of control, could coexist with an overly controlling personality. However, the connection is much deeper than it appears.

1. **Control as a coping mechanism:** Addiction often stems from a need to escape uncomfortable emotions such as fear, anxiety, or trauma. For some, controlling every aspect of their life is a way to manage these feelings, although this intense need for control can become overwhelming. When individuals can no longer control their internal world, they may turn to addictive behaviours as a way to numb or distract

themselves. In this sense, addiction can be seen as an attempt to control emotions that feel otherwise unmanageable.

2. **The illusion of control in addiction:** Addictive behaviours can create a false sense of control. For instance, a person addicted to alcohol may believe that drinking helps them 'cope' or 'manage' their stress. In reality, addiction often exacerbates the very issues it promises to solve. Despite this, the individual clings to the addictive behaviour because, on some level, it feels like control - an attempt to regulate the emotional chaos beneath the surface.

3. **Perfectionism and control:** Perfectionism is another trait closely linked to both control and addiction. Many perfectionists feel an overwhelming need to control every detail of their lives, from their work to their relationships. This can lead to immense pressure, creating feelings of inadequacy and anxiety when they inevitably fall short of impossible standards. Addiction can then emerge as a way to manage the emotional toll of striving for perfection.

4. **Emotional suppression:** Both control and addiction are methods of emotional suppression. Rather than confronting difficult feelings like shame, anger, or sadness, controlling individuals might try to structure their lives so that those emotions never surface. Although, when life becomes too chaotic to control, addiction may step in as a way to further suppress those emotions.

Why over-control happens

Several underlying psychological and emotional factors contribute to the development of controlling behaviours, particularly when they intersect with addiction:

1. **Early life experiences:** Many overly controlling individuals come from backgrounds where chaos or unpredictability was prevalent. This could include growing up in an unstable household or experiencing trauma. As a response, they develop a hypervigilant need to control everything around them to feel safe. Addiction might then arise as an escape from the relentless pressure of maintaining that control.

2. **Low self-esteem:** Often, people who need to control everything do so because they lack confidence in their own worth. By controlling their environment, they believe they can hide their vulnerabilities and inadequacies. Addiction becomes a way to self-medicate the deep-seated feelings of inadequacy.

3. **Fear of failure:** Control-oriented individuals frequently fear failure or making mistakes. The fear becomes so overwhelming that they adopt rigid patterns of behaviour, avoiding any situation where they might feel out of control. Addiction can develop as a way to manage the pressure or failure when it occurs, providing temporary relief from their self-imposed expectations.

Breaking the cycle of control and addiction

The connection between control and addiction can create a self-perpetuating cycle. As the need for control intensifies, addiction worsens, and as addiction escalates, the individual's sense of control continues to erode. Understanding this dynamic is the first step in breaking free from its grasp.

1. **Recognise the patterns:** Awareness is crucial. Those who are struggling with both control and addiction need to acknowledge the patterns they have developed. Identifying

situations where the need for control becomes overwhelming and recognising how addictive behaviours may follow are key to initiating change.

2. **Practise letting go:** One of the most important lessons for those caught in this cycle is learning how to let go of control. This does not mean becoming passive or indifferent; it is rather, recognising that some things in life are beyond our influence. This can be incredibly challenging for someone accustomed to controlling everything, yet it is vital for recovery.

3. **Develop emotional intelligence:** Both control and addiction often stem from an inability to deal with difficult emotions. Building emotional intelligence - the ability to identify, understand, and manage emotions - can help individuals navigate their feelings without resorting to control or addictive behaviours. Techniques such as mindfulness, journaling, or therapy can assist in this process.

4. **Set healthy boundaries:** Overly controlling individuals often struggle with boundaries - either imposing them too rigidly or failing to establish them at all. In recovery, learning to set healthy, flexible boundaries with oneself and others is essential. This means knowing when to take responsibility and when to allow others to act on their own.

5. **Seek professional help:** For many, breaking the cycle of control and addiction will require professional support. Therapy, particularly cognitive behavioural therapy (CBT) and dialectical behaviour therapy (DBT), can be effective in addressing both control issues and addiction. In some cases, group therapy or 12-step programmes can also provide valuable peer support.

When to seek help

Identifying when control is damaging areas of your life and is hiding addictive behaviours is crucial for early intervention. Over-controlling behaviours can obscure the underlying causes of addiction, making it difficult to recognise when professional help is needed. Here are key signs that it's time to seek support:

1. **The need for control is damaging relationships or work performance:** If controlling behaviours are straining personal relationships or affecting job performance, it's a sign that control is negatively impacting life. This can lead to isolation and professional setbacks, indicating the need for external support.

2. **The addiction is affecting physical or mental health:** When addiction worsens physical or mental health despite attempts to control it, it's time to seek professional help. The longer control is attempted without success, the more damaging the addiction becomes, potentially leading to serious health consequences.

3. **Attempts to 'manage' addiction with increased control are failing:** If trying to control or restrict addictive behaviours only results in failure, the cycle of control and addiction deepens. This failure to manage addiction through control highlights the need for effective therapeutic intervention.

4. **Increased emotional volatility:** Frequent outbursts of anger, anxiety, or frustration are often signs that the desire for control has become overwhelming. When emotional regulation begins to unravel, it can intensify addictive behaviours. Recognising this instability is crucial - it's a signal that support may be needed to regain balance and manage emotions in a healthier, more sustainable way.

Recognising these signs early allows individuals to take proactive steps towards recovery. Addressing the destructive cycle of control and addiction sooner can prevent further harm and promote healthier ways of managing emotions and behaviours.

My personal experience

The need to control every aspect of work and life contributed heavily to my exhaustion. Holding tightly to outcomes or routines drained my energy and increased stress. Learning to loosen this grip, go with the flow of life, and accept uncertainty opened up space for greater ease and allowed my wellbeing to improve. It is something that has certainly served me well and continues to do so. I will happily help others, if they are willing to help themselves. Once I realised that I couldn't do everything for everyone and that they needed to do some things for themselves, life was a lot easier, and happier. That boundary gave me the space to be present for myself and my family again.

Conclusion

The relationship between control and addiction is complex; however, understanding it can illuminate why breaking free from addiction requires addressing both the addictive behaviour and the underlying need for control. Those caught in the cycle often feel trapped between their need for order and the chaos addiction brings. With the right tools, they can regain balance.

By recognising the emotional drivers behind the need to control, practising letting go, and seeking the right support, it is possible not only to break the grip of addiction but also to develop healthier, more adaptive ways of living. Control, when balanced and flexible, can be a positive force in life. When rigid or excessive, it becomes just another form of addiction - one that, like all addictions, can be overcome.

CHAPTER 24

THE CONNECTION BETWEEN ADDICTION AND MONEY

Addiction and money are intertwined in complex ways that can often drive an individual deeper into the cycle of dependency. The connection between addiction and finances is not only about the direct costs associated with obtaining substances or engaging in addictive behaviours; it is also about how addiction affects one's financial decision-making, stability, and overall quality of life. Understanding the ways money influences addiction, and vice versa, is critical in developing effective interventions and strategies for recovery.

The connection between money and addiction

The relationship between addiction and money is a complex cycle where financial resources often fuel addictive behaviours, while addiction in turn disrupts financial stability. Whether through the cost of sustaining the addiction, impaired decision-making, or the economic consequences of lost income, money and addiction become deeply intertwined. Understanding this connection is key to addressing both the root causes and the resulting challenges individuals face.

How addiction and money intersect

At its core, addiction fundamentally alters one's priorities and decision-making processes. For many, addictive behaviours - whether related to substances like alcohol or drugs, or behaviours such as gambling, shopping, or even gaming - become the centre of focus. Financial resources, which would otherwise be used for essential living costs, savings, or future investments, are often redirected towards sustaining the addiction. This shift creates a vicious cycle: the more money is spent on the addiction, the more financial problems arise, leading to stress and, in many cases, further reliance on the addictive substance or behaviour as a coping mechanism.

Several key mechanisms demonstrate how addiction and finances intertwine:

1. **Direct costs:** Addictions are often expensive. Substances such as alcohol, drugs, or nicotine, as well as behavioural addictions like gambling or shopping, can be financially draining. The repeated need to fund these habits can lead to significant debt, the depletion of savings, or even criminal activities to obtain money.

2. **Impaired judgement:** Addiction affects the brain's reward system and impairs judgement. Individuals with addiction may not be able to consider the long-term financial consequences of their actions. The desire for immediate gratification becomes so overwhelming that they may use their rent money for a fix or gamble away their entire paycheque in the hope of a win.

3. **Loss of income and employment:** Over time, addiction can affect work performance, leading to absenteeism, decreased productivity, or even job loss. Without a steady

source of income, financial problems worsen, and the individual may feel trapped, with the addiction offering the only perceived escape.

Understanding these mechanisms is crucial for addressing the ways in which addiction and money interact, as they form the basis for the connection's persistence and intensity. Without intervention, these patterns become deeply entrenched, creating both economic and emotional barriers to recovery.

Why there is a connection between addiction and money

Addiction and money are closely linked due to the way addiction prioritises immediate gratification over long-term financial wellbeing. This relationship is influenced by psychological, social, and economic factors, where money often becomes either a means to sustain addiction or a source of stress. There are several reasons why addiction and money are so closely linked:

1. **Immediate reward vs. long-term gain:** Addictions exploit the brain's reward pathways, prioritising immediate pleasure over long-term wellbeing. In financial terms, this translates to spending money impulsively for the instant 'high' or temporary relief, rather than saving or investing for future stability.

2. **Escapism:** Many individuals turn to addiction as a means to escape their problems, including financial stress. Paradoxically, the very behaviour used to escape financial worries often exacerbates the situation, leading to a cycle of increasing dependency and mounting debt.

3. **Social and environmental factors:** In some communities,

poverty and financial instability may increase the risk of addiction. Economic hardship can create an environment where individuals seek comfort or an escape from reality, often through substances or behaviours that can provide temporary relief. Additionally, individuals in these environments may lack the financial education or resources necessary to manage money responsibly, further compounding their risk of addiction.

How this connection happens

The connection between addiction and finances is driven by biological, psychological, and societal factors that reinforce each other. These influences affect decision-making and behaviour, making it difficult for individuals to break the cycle. Several factors play a role in forming and maintaining the link between addiction and finances:

1. **Biological factors:** Addiction affects the brain's reward circuitry and decision-making processes. As a result, individuals may become preoccupied with short-term gains (e.g., the immediate pleasure from drugs or gambling wins) at the expense of long-term consequences, including financial ruin.

2. **Psychological factors:** For many, addiction stems from underlying psychological issues such as stress, anxiety, or trauma. The relief provided by substances or addictive behaviours can be so powerful that financial consequences seem inconsequential. As the addiction progresses, money becomes a means to an end - a tool to maintain access to the substance or behaviour rather than a resource to manage one's life.

3. **Cultural and societal influences:** Society often promotes instant gratification, materialism, and consumption, creating environments where spending and indulgence are encouraged. For those struggling with addiction, this societal pressure can intensify the relationship between their behaviour and financial choices, reinforcing the cycle.

What to do

Addressing the connection between addiction and finances requires a multi-faceted approach that targets both the addiction itself and the financial behaviours associated with it. Below are several steps and strategies:

1. **Financial education and counselling:** Financial education can play a significant role in breaking the cycle of addiction and financial mismanagement. Learning about budgeting, saving, and debt management empowers individuals to make better financial decisions. Coupled with addiction counselling, this approach can help individuals recognise the impact of their spending and develop healthier habits.

2. **Setting up boundaries:** In cases where individuals struggle to manage their money while dealing with addiction, it may be helpful for them to set up financial boundaries. This could mean having a trusted friend or family member manage their finances temporarily, establishing strict budgets, or limiting access to cash and credit cards.

3. **Seeking professional help:** Addiction is a complex condition that often requires professional intervention. Addiction treatment programmes, whether outpatient or residential, can provide structured environments where individuals can begin to manage their finances alongside their recovery.

This may include therapy sessions focused on developing coping mechanisms that do not involve spending or substances.

4. **Debt relief and financial assistance programmes:** For those already facing severe financial consequences, seeking debt relief services or financial assistance programmes can be beneficial. These services can help restructure debt and provide a path toward financial recovery, reducing the immediate stressors that might trigger addictive behaviours.

When to seek help

Recognising the right time to address the connection between addiction and money is crucial for effective intervention. Early intervention can prevent further financial and emotional damage, making it easier to break the cycle of addiction. Key indicators that it may be time to take action include:

1. **Escalating debt or inability to pay bills:** If addiction has led to significant debt or an inability to meet basic financial obligations, seeking help immediately is critical. The longer these financial issues persist, the harder it becomes to regain control over both finances and the addiction itself. Unmanaged debt can quickly become overwhelming, leading to long-term consequences like bankruptcy or foreclosure.

2. **Job loss or decreased income:** A loss of employment due to addiction, or a noticeable decline in work performance, signals the need for immediate intervention. Without a stable income, financial instability will likely worsen, further fuelling the addiction. Recovery from both the addiction and its financial impact becomes much harder without stable

employment or income to support the process.

3. **Legal or criminal consequences:** In some cases, the need for money to sustain an addiction can lead individuals to engage in illegal activities, such as theft, fraud, or other criminal behaviours. If addiction has progressed to this point, urgent professional assistance is needed to address both the legal and addiction issues. Criminal charges not only add to the financial burden; they can also create long-term consequences that complicate recovery.

Taking action at these critical points can prevent further escalation and create a stronger foundation for recovery, both financially and personally. The earlier support is sought, the more likely it is to break the damaging cycle of addiction and financial instability.

My personal experience

As a husband and father, providing for my family has always been my priority, ensuring that they have enough of whatever they need, and that they are always cared for and protected. This need to earn money has always driven me to work for longer and harder than I perhaps should have, even if I do enjoy what I do. Wealth to me is not only centred around money, it also includes balance, relationships, personal enjoyment, achievements – things for a time I had undervalued.

Conclusion

The relationship between addiction and money is deeply rooted in the biological, psychological, and social fabric of addiction itself. Understanding this connection is crucial for developing effective strategies to combat addiction and promote financial stability. Financial counselling, addiction treatment, and support networks are key components in addressing the intertwined issues of money and addiction. By addressing both the psychological aspects of addiction and the practical, financial habits that sustain it, individuals can begin to rebuild their lives, achieving both recovery and financial security.

CHAPTER 25

THE CONNECTION BETWEEN ADDICTION AND STRESS

Addiction is often thought of as a standalone condition, tied solely to the substance or behaviour at hand. However, it is far more complex. One significant factor that can drive or exacerbate addiction is stress. Stress, in its many forms, plays a critical role in both the onset of addictive behaviours and the challenges faced in recovery. This chapter will explore the intricate relationship between stress and addiction, addressing how stress fuels addiction, why this connection exists, and what steps can be taken to manage it effectively.

The connection between stress and addiction

Stress is a natural response to external pressures or threats, whether physical, emotional, or psychological. It triggers the body's 'fight-or-flight' response, releasing hormones like cortisol and adrenaline to help us cope. While this response is useful in short bursts, chronic stress can lead to adverse mental and physical health outcomes, including addiction.

As we have seen in earlier chapters, addiction is often seen as an attempt to self-medicate – a way for individuals to cope with overwhelming feelings or experiences. When someone is under stress, their brain craves relief. Substances like alcohol or drugs, or behaviours such as gambling or overeating, can provide temporary respite by affecting the brain's reward system. Over time, this cycle of stress-relief-reward can evolve into addiction.

Why it happens

Stress affects the brain's prefrontal cortex, which is responsible for decision-making and impulse control. Under prolonged stress, the brain's ability to regulate these functions becomes impaired, making it harder for individuals to resist temptation or make sound decisions. The limbic system, which governs emotional responses and pleasure-seeking, can dominate, driving a person to seek out unhealthy coping mechanisms to alleviate stress.

Types of stress that contribute to addiction

Stress comes in many forms, each with the potential to increase the risk of addiction:

1. **Acute stress:** Sudden or short-term stress, such as a job loss or a death in the family, can trigger addictive behaviours as a quick way to numb the emotional pain.

2. **Chronic stress:** Ongoing stress, like financial difficulties or relationship problems, wears down the body's defences over time, making it easier to succumb to addictive habits.

3. **Traumatic stress:** Experiencing trauma, especially in childhood (e.g., abuse or neglect), can deeply affect how a person copes with stress as an adult. Many individuals with addiction have a history of trauma, and their substance or behavioural dependencies often serve as a way to escape unresolved emotions.

4. **Occupational stress:** Stress related to work can also contribute to addiction. High-pressure jobs, long hours, or a toxic work environment can leave people seeking an outlet through substances or addictive behaviours like gambling or smoking.

Why stress is such a powerful trigger

The neurochemical changes that occur during periods of stress are key to understanding why it can trigger addiction. Under stress, the brain's reward system becomes more sensitive to the effects of addictive substances or activities. Dopamine, the neurotransmitter associated with pleasure and reward, is released in higher quantities when a person engages in addictive behaviour. This creates a powerful feedback loop where the brain links stress relief with the addictive substance or behaviour.

Over time, tolerance develops, requiring more of the substance or activity to achieve the same level of stress relief. This is why stress is not just a trigger for addiction; it can also reinforce and deepen it. For someone already struggling with addiction, stress makes it even more difficult to abstain, as the brain begins to prioritise immediate relief over long-term wellbeing.

The vicious cycle of stress and addiction

Addiction often worsens stress in the long run, creating a vicious cycle. Initially, addictive behaviours may offer short-term relief. However, as dependence grows, the consequences of addiction – such as financial strain, relationship issues, or health problems – add to the person's overall stress. This, in turn, drives them back to the substance or behaviour as a way to cope, reinforcing the cycle of addiction.

For instance, someone who drinks alcohol to relax after a stressful day may feel temporary relief. However, the following morning, they may experience physical symptoms of a hangover, regret their actions, or face criticism from loved ones, adding to their stress. They then turn to alcohol again to numb these negative feelings, thus perpetuating the cycle.

Strategies for breaking the stress–addiction cycle

Understanding the connection between stress and addiction is the first step towards recovery. The next is identifying effective ways to manage stress without resorting to addictive behaviours. Here are some key strategies for breaking the cycle:

1. **Recognising triggers:** It's crucial to recognise what triggers you to experience stress and, by extension, your addictive behaviour. Keeping a stress journal can help you identify patterns, situations, or people that tend to increase your stress levels. Once you understand your triggers, you can take steps to either avoid them or develop healthier ways to respond to them.

2. **Mindfulness and relaxation techniques:** Mindfulness practices, such as meditation, deep breathing exercises, and progressive muscle relaxation, can help reduce the impact of stress. By staying present and focusing on your breathing or bodily sensations, you can break the cycle of stress before it escalates into an addictive behaviour. Regular practice of these techniques helps build resilience to stress over time.

3. **Physical activity:** Exercise is one of the most effective ways to combat stress. Physical activity releases endorphins, the brain's natural mood boosters, and can help restore balance to your body's stress hormones. Even light exercises, like

walking, swimming, or yoga, can significantly reduce stress levels and improve overall wellbeing.

4. **Social support:** Isolation often exacerbates both stress and addiction. Seeking support from friends, family, or support groups can help reduce feelings of stress and loneliness. Talking to someone who understands your struggles can offer new perspectives on dealing with stress without resorting to addictive behaviour.

5. **Cognitive behavioural therapy (CBT):** CBT is particularly effective in addressing the relationship between stress and addiction. CBT can help you identify negative thought patterns, develop coping mechanisms, and replace unhealthy responses with more productive ones. CBT can also help address underlying issues, such as trauma, that may be contributing to both stress and addiction.

6. **Healthy routine:** Establishing a structured daily routine can provide stability and predictability, which reduces stress. By creating a schedule that includes time for self-care, exercise, relaxation, and social interaction, you can reduce the likelihood of stress triggering addictive behaviours.

When to seek help

Recognising when stress has become overwhelming and is driving addictive behaviours is vital for maintaining mental and physical wellbeing. If stress has escalated to a point where it feels uncontrollable and is leading you toward or deepening addictive behaviours, professional help may be necessary. The following signs can help identify when it's time to seek support:

1. **Feeling overwhelmed by stress on a daily basis:** If stress

becomes a constant presence in your life, leaving you feeling overwhelmed every day, it may be a sign that it has reached an unmanageable level. Chronic stress can erode your coping mechanisms, increasing the likelihood of turning to substances or addictive behaviours for relief.

2. **Using substances or addictive behaviours more frequently or in larger quantities:** Turning to alcohol, drugs, or other addictive activities as a way to cope with stress is common; however, when the frequency or intensity of these behaviours increases, it signals that stress is driving dependence. Using more of a substance, or engaging in a behaviour more often, in an attempt to manage stress, is a clear indicator that control is slipping.

3. **Experiencing withdrawal symptoms when not engaging in the addictive behaviour:** Withdrawal symptoms - whether physical or psychological - when not engaging in the addictive behaviour, such as irritability, anxiety, or cravings, are red flags. This shows that your body and mind have become reliant on the substance or behaviour as a stress-relief mechanism.

4. **Noticing a significant impact on health, relationships, or work:** If the stress-induced addictive behaviour is affecting your physical health, damaging relationships, or impairing your work or studies, it's a strong sign that intervention is needed. These negative impacts on your life can escalate and worsen the cycle of addiction, making it more difficult to break free without professional assistance.

Acting early by reaching out for help can significantly improve the chances of long-term recovery and restore your ability to manage stress healthily without relying on addictive behaviours.

My personal experience

I remember always feeling as if I had a spinning motor inside of me, like a catherine wheel on fireworks night, going at 100 MPH. I was constantly on high alert and stress was my unrelenting companion. However, underneath that busyness were burnout, anxiety, and avoidance. Stress was both the trigger and the excuse – a reason to push harder, to do more, to keep moving forward. Rainford Hall taught me the value of rest, not as a reward, but as a necessity. That change in mind-set has been transformative for me.

Conclusion

Stress and addiction are deeply intertwined, each feeding off the other in a destructive cycle. However, understanding this connection opens the door to recovery. By recognising the role of stress in addiction and implementing effective stress management techniques, individuals can break free from the hold of addiction. Learning to cope with stress in healthier ways is a fundamental step on the journey to long-lasting recovery, allowing individuals to regain control of their lives and embrace a future free from addiction.

CHAPTER 26

THE CONNECTION BETWEEN ADDICTION AND TRAUMA

Trauma and addiction are intricately connected, creating a complex and deeply intertwined relationship that can shape an individual's mental, emotional, and physical wellbeing over the course of their life. Trauma, whether experienced during childhood or adulthood, often leaves deep psychological scars that can influence coping mechanisms and behaviours. Addiction, in many cases, emerges as a way to self-soothe or escape from the overwhelming pain and distress caused by traumatic experiences.

The connection between trauma and addiction

Trauma and addiction are linked through both biological and psychological pathways. When individuals experience trauma, their nervous systems can remain in a heightened state of stress for prolonged periods. The body releases stress hormones like cortisol and adrenaline, which can become dysregulated, affecting mood, energy levels, and the ability to cope.

Addictive substances or behaviours may provide a temporary escape from these overwhelming emotions. For example:

1. **Self-medication hypothesis:** Individuals may use substances[hmmm] to numb emotional pain, alleviate anxiety, or combat feelings of worthlessness stemming from trauma.

2. **Dopamine dysregulation:** Trauma can impair the brain's reward system, making it harder for individuals to feel pleasure. Drugs and alcohol artificially stimulate dopamine release, providing a fleeting sense of relief.

3. **Coping mechanisms:** Trauma survivors often lack healthy coping strategies due to disrupted development or lack of support. Addiction can serve as a maladaptive although accessible way to manage distress.

How trauma affects vulnerability to addiction

Trauma-informed care addresses both trauma and addiction by creating safety, building trust, empowering individuals, and avoiding re-traumatisation, supporting effective recovery and healing.

1. **Neurological changes:** Chronic trauma can lead to alterations in brain structures like the amygdala, prefrontal cortex, and hippocampus. These changes increase vulnerability to addiction by heightening emotional reactivity and impairing decision-making.

2. **Attachment issues:** Traumatic experiences, especially in childhood, can disrupt the formation of secure attachments. Individuals with insecure or disorganised attachment styles are more likely to seek external sources of comfort, such as illegal substances or alcohol.

3. **Mental health co-morbidities:** Trauma often leads to mental health conditions like post-traumatic stress disorder (PTSD), depression, or anxiety. These conditions

significantly increase the risk of developing an addiction.

4. **Social and environmental factors:** A history of trauma often coincides with social instability, poverty, or lack of access to mental health care, all of which can exacerbate addiction risk.

Why the connection matters

The relationship between trauma and addiction is significant because it underscores the necessity of addressing both issues simultaneously for meaningful and lasting recovery. Trauma often serves as a root cause of addiction, with individuals using substances to self-medicate and numb the pain of unresolved experiences. However, without addressing the underlying trauma, addiction recovery efforts can be incomplete or short-lived, as the driving forces behind the behaviour remain unexamined and untreated.

Trauma-informed care (see below) is critical in this context, as it provides a framework that prioritises the individual's safety, trust, and empowerment. This approach recognises that traditional treatment methods can inadvertently re-traumatise individuals, impeding their progress. Instead, trauma-informed care integrates an understanding of trauma's impact on every aspect of treatment, creating an environment that supports healing on both emotional and behavioural levels. This holistic approach enables individuals to confront and process their trauma while building the tools they need to sustain sobriety.

How to address trauma and addiction

Trauma-informed care: As already described, trauma-informed care emphasises a compassionate, patient-centred approach that acknowledges the profound effects of trauma on an individual's behaviour and psyche. Core principles of trauma-informed care include:

1. **Creating a safe environment:** Establishing both physical and emotional safety is foundational. Treatment settings should be free of judgement, ensure confidentiality, and foster a sense of comfort and stability. For trauma survivors, feeling safe is the first step toward building trust and engaging in recovery.

2. **Building trust:** Trust is cultivated through transparent communication, consistent actions, and respecting the individual's boundaries. A predictable and reliable approach helps create a sense of security, enabling individuals to open up and participate fully in the healing process.

3. **Empowering clients:** Empowerment involves helping individuals regain control over their lives by involving them in decision-making processes. This might include collaborating on treatment goals, offering choices, and recognising their strengths and resilience. Empowerment fosters self-efficacy and a sense of autonomy.

4. **Avoiding re-traumatisation:** Practitioners must be mindful of language, practices, or interventions that could inadvertently trigger traumatic memories. This includes avoiding confrontational techniques, maintaining a calm and supportive tone, and tailoring treatment to the individual's comfort level.

Therapies for trauma and addiction

Several evidence-based therapies have proven effective in addressing both trauma and addiction. These therapies are designed to help individuals process their traumatic experiences, develop healthier coping mechanisms, and break free from the cycle of substance misuse. Some of the most well-established therapies include:

1. **Cognitive behavioural therapy (CBT):** CBT is a structured, goal-oriented therapy that helps individuals identify and challenge negative thought patterns related to trauma and addiction. It equips them with practical strategies to manage triggers, cope with cravings, and develop healthier behaviours.

2. **Eye movement desensitisation and reprocessing (EMDR):** EMDR is a specialised therapy designed to process and reframe traumatic memories. By using bilateral stimulation (such as guided eye movements), EMDR helps reduce the emotional impact of trauma, enabling individuals to reprocess their experiences in a less distressing way.

3. **Somatic experiencing:** This body-focused therapy addresses the physical manifestations of trauma, such as chronic tension or hyperarousal. By working with the body's natural responses, somatic experiencing helps individuals release stored trauma and restore a sense of physical and emotional balance.

4. **Group therapy:** Group therapy provides a sense of community, normalising the individual's experiences and fostering connection with others who have faced similar challenges. This shared support can be particularly healing for trauma survivors who feel isolated or misunderstood.

5. **Medication-assisted treatment (MAT):** For individuals struggling with trauma-related addiction, medication can sometimes play a supportive role. Antidepressants,

anti-anxiety medications, or medications like naltrexone and buprenorphine can help manage symptoms and reduce cravings, complementing therapeutic interventions.

Building resilience

Resilience is the ability to adapt, recover, and grow stronger in the face of adversity. For trauma survivors, building resilience is a vital part of the healing process. Strategies include:

1. **Mindfulness and meditation:** Mindfulness practices enhance present-moment awareness and reduce emotional reactivity. Techniques like deep breathing, meditation, or yoga can help individuals develop a greater sense of calm and control.

2. **Support networks:** Connection with supportive friends, family members, or peer groups can offer encouragement and a sense of belonging. Support networks provide a vital buffer against isolation and foster accountability during recovery.

3. **Healthy lifestyle choices:** Physical health and mental wellbeing are closely linked, as we have seen. Encouraging regular exercise, balanced nutrition, and adequate sleep helps individuals build strength and resilience, improving their capacity to cope with challenges.

4. **Setting goals:** Helping individuals set small, manageable goals can rebuild confidence and a sense of purpose. Each achievement reinforces their progress and motivates them to continue on their recovery journey.

When to seek help

Early intervention is essential to breaking the cycle of trauma and addiction. Recognising warning signs enables timely support and reduces the risk of further harm. Key indicators include:

1. **Substance use as a coping mechanism:** If individuals are using drugs or alcohol to numb emotions, escape painful memories, or manage anxiety, it is a clear signal that intervention may be needed.

2. **Recurrent relapse:** Persistent difficulties in maintaining sobriety/abstinence often point to unresolved trauma. Relapse (see Chapter 10) can signify that deeper emotional wounds require attention before sustainable recovery is possible.

3. **Behavioural changes:** Withdrawal from loved ones, increased irritability, or engagement in risky behaviours may signal underlying trauma. Such changes should prompt concern and exploration of their root causes.

4. **Mental health symptoms:** Anxiety, depression, or symptoms of PTSD that accompany or precede addiction are key red flags. Addressing these mental health challenges alongside addiction is crucial for holistic recovery.

Timely intervention should focus on integrated care that addresses both trauma and addiction simultaneously. By providing comprehensive support, it is possible to break the cycle, foster healing, and help individuals build a healthier and more fulfilling life.

My personal experience

I've experienced my fair share of personal traumas, as you'll discover - and perhaps reflect on in relation to your own experiences - in my background story at the end of this book (see page 447). These include long-standing challenges such as my parents' divorce when I was around seven, my siblings' personal struggles, and illness that led to me having 45 operations before the age of 16. Alongside these came specific near-death events that profoundly shaped my outlook on life and contributed to my pushing myself to near breaking point. I am deeply grateful to my wife and my brother for helping me see the reality of my situation and guiding me back onto a healthier path, along with the timely and transformative support I received from Rainford Hall (see page xi).

Conclusion

The connection between trauma and addiction is profound, with trauma leaving an indelible mark on the brain, body, and spirit. These experiences create vulnerabilities that often lead individuals to seek relief through addictive behaviours, as substances or compulsive actions may temporarily numb emotional pain or anxiety. The disrupted brain chemistry caused by trauma can make addiction harder to overcome, as recovery requires addressing not just the addictive behaviours but also the underlying psychological wounds. Understanding this intricate relationship is key to effective treatment, which must be trauma-informed, prioritising safety, trust, and empowerment in the healing process.

Recovery is possible when individuals are provided with the right tools, support, and understanding. It is not just about overcoming addiction; it is also about healing the deeper emotional and psychological scars left by trauma. A holistic approach, integrating therapies, community support, and resilience-building techniques, can help individuals rebuild their sense of self, regain control over their lives, and develop healthier coping strategies. With the right resources, individuals can not only recover from addiction; they can also reclaim their lives, experiencing renewed purpose, well-being, and strength.

CHAPTER 27

THE CONNECTION BETWEEN ADDICTION AND RELATIONSHIPS

Addiction, at its core, is a deeply personal experience. However, its ripple effects extend far beyond the individual, often reaching into the very fabric of their relationships. As addiction takes hold, relationships - whether familial, romantic, or social - become entangled in the complexities of this struggle. Addiction can act as both a cause and a consequence within relationships, altering dynamics and causing significant harm. This chapter seeks to unravel the intricate connection between addiction and relationships, exploring how addiction influences relational patterns, why these links form, and what can be done to break free from destructive cycles and build healthier, more supportive bonds.

The connection between relationships and addiction

Human beings are inherently social creatures, reliant on relationships for emotional security, validation, and support. However, these same relationships can sometimes foster unhealthy dynamics, particularly when addiction is at play. The connection between addiction and relationships is shaped by several key factors that intertwine in ways that can be difficult to untangle:

1. **Emotional escapism:** Many individuals turn to addictive behaviours as a way to cope with the pain of strained relationships. Whether the issues stem from unresolved conflicts, feelings of inadequacy, emotional neglect, or loneliness, addiction often offers a temporary reprieve from the overwhelming discomfort of relational distress. The addictive behaviour becomes a way to numb emotions and avoid facing difficult truths or difficult conversations.

2. **Co-dependency:** Addiction can foster co-dependent relationships, where one partner - knowingly or unknowingly - enables the other's addictive behaviours. In this dynamic, the enabler may feel validated or necessary by taking on the role of 'caretaker' or 'protector', while the addict becomes dependent on the enabler to avoid facing the natural consequences of their addiction. This unbalanced relationship allows the cycle of addiction to continue unchecked, with both parties becoming stuck in a toxic loop.

3. **Shared environments:** Addiction doesn't just affect the individual; it can spread within social circles, family units, or romantic partnerships, especially when addictive behaviours become normalised within these environments. In some groups, behaviours like excessive drinking or drug use may be casually accepted as part of social interactions. When these behaviours are normalised or even celebrated, it becomes more difficult for individuals to resist or break free from the addictive patterns that develop within these shared environments.

4. **Childhood influences:** Dysfunctional family dynamics, such as neglect, abuse, or inconsistent parenting, often lay the groundwork for relational and addictive struggles in adulthood. These early-life experiences shape attachment

styles, emotional regulation, and coping mechanisms. Individuals who experienced trauma or neglect in childhood may be predisposed to addiction and relational dependency, as they often struggle to form healthy, secure attachments and may turn to addictive substances or behaviours to manage their emotional pain.

5. **Trauma bonds:** Some relationships, particularly those built on shared trauma or unhealed emotional wounds, can create a bond that is both powerful and unhealthy. Addiction may act as the common ground that sustains these relationships, even though the addiction itself perpetuates harm. In these cases, individuals may find it difficult to leave or break free from toxic relational patterns, as the bond formed through shared pain can feel intensely binding and all-consuming.

How addiction affects relationships

Addiction has far-reaching consequences for relationships, often causing a cycle of dysfunction and emotional pain. The most common effects of addiction on relationships include:

1. **Erosion of trust:** Addictive behaviours are often accompanied by secrecy, dishonesty, and betrayal. Whether it's hiding the extent of the addiction, lying about substance use, or betraying a partner's trust in other ways, addiction causes a breakdown in the foundation of trust that relationships rely on. Over time, these betrayals create deep emotional wounds that are difficult to heal, leaving lasting scars on both the addict and their loved ones.

2. **Emotional distance:** Addiction tends to turn the focus of the addicted individual inward, making them less emotionally

available to their partner, family, or friends. As the addiction takes priority, the addict becomes increasingly absorbed in their own internal world, leaving loved ones feeling neglected, emotionally abandoned, and unimportant. This emotional distance creates a sense of isolation within the relationship, often leading to feelings of rejection and heartache for those who care about the addict.

3. **Conflict and resentment:** The financial strain, erratic behaviour, and unmet expectations that often accompany addiction lead to frequent conflicts and growing resentment. As addiction takes hold, partners, family members, and friends may become frustrated and angry by the addict's inability or unwillingness to change. This simmering resentment can result in constant arguments and a deterioration of the relationship, with both sides feeling misunderstood and unsupported.

4. **Role reversals:** In some relationships, one partner or family member may assume a caregiving or protective role due to the addict's behaviour. This shift can create unhealthy power dynamics, with the caregiver taking on the burden of managing the addict's issues, often at the expense of their own emotional wellbeing. Over time, this role reversal can lead to burnout, resentment, and a sense of emotional disconnection, as the caregiving partner feels trapped in a role they didn't choose.

5. **Isolation:** Addicts may withdraw from healthy relationships due to feelings of shame, guilt, or the isolating nature of their addiction. In some cases, the addict's withdrawal is a self-protective measure to avoid facing the consequences of their behaviour. Conversely, loved ones may also distance themselves out of frustration, self-preservation, or a lack of

understanding of how to help. This mutual isolation only worsens the emotional strain, leaving both the addict and their loved ones feeling unsupported and alone.

How this connection happens

The intricate connection between addiction and relationships is often rooted in psychological and physiological mechanisms that impact both individuals and their interactions:

1. **Reward systems:** Addiction hijacks the brain's reward system, prioritising the addictive substance or behaviour over all else, including relationships. The brain releases dopamine in response to the addictive activity, creating feelings of pleasure and reinforcing the desire to repeat the behaviour. As the addiction takes hold, the addict becomes increasingly focused on satisfying their cravings, often at the expense of their relational connections.

2. **Attachment styles:** People with insecure attachment styles - whether anxious, avoidant, or disorganised - may turn to addiction as a way of coping with relational fears such as abandonment, rejection, or intimacy. Individuals with these attachment issues may struggle to trust others or to form stable, healthy relationships. Instead of addressing their emotional needs directly, they may rely on substances or behaviours to numb the discomfort caused by relational uncertainty.

3. **Stress and coping:** High levels of stress, whether from external pressures or relational strife, can push individuals towards addiction as a maladaptive coping mechanism. When faced with difficult life circumstances or relationship challenges, some individuals may turn to

drugs, alcohol, or other addictive behaviours to temporarily escape their stress or emotional pain. Unfortunately, these behaviours only serve to intensify the underlying issues, exacerbating the cycle of addiction and relational dysfunction.

4. **Patterns of enmeshment:** In some relationships, individuals become so enmeshed that their identities and emotional needs are inseparable. This lack of healthy boundaries can foster environments where addiction thrives, as both individuals struggle to maintain their sense of self while navigating the challenges of the addiction. This enmeshment can create a co-dependent or toxic dynamic in which addiction becomes the focal point of the relationship, preventing both partners from developing the autonomy and emotional health needed to heal.

What can be done to break the cycle

Breaking the cycle of addiction and relational dysfunction requires a holistic, multi-faceted approach that involves personal healing, relational repair, and systemic changes. Some key strategies for breaking the cycle include:

1. **Seek professional help:** Therapy, whether individual or couples' counselling, can provide a safe space to address the underlying issues driving both addiction and relational problems.

2. **Set boundaries:** Establishing clear boundaries is essential for breaking cycles of co-dependency and enabling. This might include refusing to cover up for an addict's behaviours or prioritising self-care.

3. **Foster open communication:** Honest, empathetic dialogue can help rebuild trust and address lingering resentments. Structured conversations guided by a therapist can be particularly effective.

4. **Education and awareness:** Understanding the nature of addiction can help loved ones approach the situation with compassion rather than judgement. Education can also dispel myths and reduce stigma.

5. **Engage in support networks:** Joining support groups such as Al-Anon, Families Anonymous, or similar organisations can provide guidance, validation, and a sense of community for both addicts and their loved ones.

6. **Address underlying trauma:** Addiction and relational difficulties often stem from unresolved trauma. Trauma-focused therapies (see Chapter 26), such as EMDR or somatic experiencing, can help individuals process and heal from past wounds.

7. **Promote healthy habits:** Encouraging activities that foster wellbeing, such as exercise, mindfulness, or creative pursuits, can help replace addictive behaviours and strengthen relational bonds.

When to seek help

Timing is crucial when addressing addiction within the context of relationships. Key moments to consider intervention include:

1. **Early signs of dysfunction:** Addressing issues early on, before they escalate, can prevent long-term damage. Early intervention allows individuals to confront problems before they become deeply ingrained and harder to change.

2. **Crisis points:** Major events such as a health scare, legal trouble, or financial collapse can serve as turning points for change. These moments of crisis can provide an opportunity to reassess priorities, recognise the severity of the addiction, and take action toward recovery.

3. **Readiness for change:** Interventions are most effective when the individual is ready to acknowledge their addiction and its impact on their relationships. If the person is not yet ready to face the issue, forcing intervention may only lead to resistance and further conflict.

4. **Escalation of harm:** If addiction leads to abuse, neglect, or significant harm within the relationship, immediate intervention is necessary to protect all parties involved. Ensuring safety and wellbeing should always be the top priority in situations where harm is escalating.

My personal experience

My internal exhaustion and defensiveness sometimes leaked into my interactions with others - which could have created tension or distance. At times I felt the need to wear a mask to maintain appearances or meet expectations; this saved me from answering questions I did not want to address, which in-turn prevented me from expressing my true needs. Learning to communicate openly and set boundaries was transformative. It allowed me to nurture more honest, supportive, and fulfilling relationships.

Chapter 27

Conclusion

The connection between addiction and relationships is complex, multifaceted, and deeply rooted in human behaviour and emotion. While addiction can strain even the strongest bonds, it is possible to break the cycle and foster healthier dynamics through awareness, compassion, and proactive intervention. Healing is rarely linear; however, with commitment, support, and the right strategies, individuals and their relationships can move toward a brighter, addiction-free future.

CHAPTER 28

THE CONNECTION BETWEEN ADDICTION AND FAMILY LIFE

Addiction is a deeply personal struggle, yet it rarely exists in isolation. When individuals face addiction while raising children or living within a family unit, the impact ripples far beyond the person directly involved. This chapter explores why family dynamics, particularly the presence of children, often intersect with addiction, how these relationships influence one another, and strategies for addressing this complex interplay. Understanding these connections is vital for breaking cycles of harm and building healthier futures.

The connection between family life and addiction

For parents, the stresses of caregiving, financial pressures, and unresolved personal struggles can make addictive substances or behaviours seem like an escape. Meanwhile, children often bear the emotional weight of a parent's addiction, experiencing confusion, fear, and long-term psychological effects. Understanding this interplay is essential to breaking harmful cycles, offering support to those in need, and fostering healthier, more resilient families.

Why there is a connection between addiction and family life

Addiction often stems from and feeds into emotional and psychological stressors, and the family unit can be a fertile ground for these triggers.

1. **Emotional pressures:** Parenting and maintaining a family come with immense responsibilities, from financial strain to emotional labour. For some, certain substances or behaviours become a coping mechanism for overwhelming demands. Alcohol, drugs, or addictive behaviours may seem like a quick escape from the pressures of caregiving or unresolved family conflicts.

2. **Intergenerational patterns:** Addiction may perpetuate through generations. Children raised in households with addiction are statistically more likely to develop substance abuse issues themselves. Trauma, normalisation of substance use, and/or genetic predisposition often create cycles that are challenging to break.

3. **The role of isolation:** Family life, particularly when caring for young children, can sometimes feel isolating. Parents who feel unsupported or disconnected from their communities may turn to substances or behaviours as substitutes for the connection and fulfilment they lack.

4. **Stress, conflict, and co-dependency:** Addiction can both result from and exacerbate unhealthy family dynamics. Marital conflicts, financial instability, or co-dependent relationships within the family (see page 405) often create an environment where addictive behaviours flourish.

How addiction impacts the family unit

Addiction extends beyond the individual, deeply affecting the family unit. It disrupts relationships, strains emotional bonds, and often creates financial and psychological burdens for loved ones. Understanding these impacts is essential to support both the individual in recovery and the family as a whole.

1. **Emotional effects on children:** Children are often the silent victims of addiction. Witnessing a parent or family member's struggle can lead to feelings of confusion, shame, or fear. Over time, children may internalise these experiences, manifesting in anxiety, depression, or their own addictive tendencies.

2. **Strain on relationships:** Addiction reshapes familial relationships, often creating a divide between the person struggling and their loved ones. Trust erodes, and resentment can build, resulting in strained or severed bonds.

3. **Economic and social consequences:** Addictions can drain financial resources, disrupt routines, and hinder personal and professional development, affecting the family's overall stability and wellbeing.

4. **Role reversal:** In severe cases, children may take on caregiving roles, leading to parentification. This reversal of roles places an undue burden on young minds and can result in lasting psychological scars.

Factors that make addiction more likely in a family context

Certain family dynamics, such as genetics, environmental stress, or learned behaviours, can increase the likelihood of addiction. These factors often create a cycle where addiction becomes more prevalent across generations.

1. **Unresolved trauma:** Individuals often bring their own unprocessed trauma into the family unit. Without healthy coping mechanisms or support systems, they may turn to addiction as a way to numb pain.

2. **Lack of support networks:** Families with limited access to external support, such as extended family, friends, or community services, are more vulnerable to addiction.

3. **Cultural and societal norms:** Societal pressures to appear as a 'perfect' family, or cultural acceptance of certain substances, can contribute to the problem. For instance, the normalisation of drinking alcohol at social events may mask early signs of alcohol dependency.

4. **Mental health factors:** Anxiety, depression, or other mental health issues often coexist with addiction. Parenting, which magnifies these challenges, can create a perfect storm for dependency to take hold.

What to do when addiction enters a family dynamic

Breaking free from addiction within a family context requires a dual focus: addressing the individual's addiction and mending the family unit.

1. **Recognising the problem:** The first step is acknowledging that addiction exists and understanding its impact on the family. This can be a painful process, especially when denial has been a protective shield.

2. **Seek professional help:** Therapy, whether individual,

couples, or family-based, can provide a safe space for addressing underlying issues. Rehabilitation programmes or addiction specialists may offer tailored support for the addicted individual.

3. **Establish open communication:** Transparent dialogue is essential. Family members will help the situation by striving to create an environment where feelings, frustrations, and fears can be shared without judgement.

4. **Set boundaries:** For families dealing with addiction, establishing clear boundaries is crucial. Boundaries protect children and ensure that the addicted individual is held accountable while receiving support.

5. **Provide stability for children:** Safeguarding the wellbeing of children is a top priority. Schools, community groups, or counselling services can offer additional support to help children navigate the challenges of living with addiction in the family.

6. **Educate yourself:** Understanding addiction as a disease rather than a moral failing can reduce stigma and promote empathy. Learning about the nature of addiction can empower families to respond constructively.

7. **Involving the family in recovery:** Recovery works best when the entire family participates. Family therapy can help rebuild trust, improve communication, and address underlying issues that contribute to the addiction.

8. **Prioritising self-care:** Both the person struggling with addiction and their family members need to prioritise self-care. Resilience comes from maintaining mental and physical wellbeing.

Building a healthier future

Creating a healthier future involves breaking the cycle of addiction and fostering supportive environments for recovery. This process includes addressing underlying issues, building resilience, and empowering individuals and families to make lasting, positive changes. Recovery is not just about the individual; it's a collective effort. A healthier future involves:

1. **Breaking the cycle:** Providing children with tools and education about addiction can prevent them from following similar paths. Focus on building resilience and self-esteem in children.

2. **Rebuilding trust:** Trust takes time to restore. Families are recommended to approach this process with patience, acknowledging progress rather than perfection.

3. **Fostering connection:** Strong, supportive relationships within the family can help prevent relapse and promote long-term wellbeing.

4. **Celebrating milestones:** Acknowledge and celebrate the victories, however small. Recovery is a journey, and recognising progress reinforces hope and motivation.

When to seek help

Addressing addiction within a family requires careful timing and observation. The earlier help is sought, the more likely it is to prevent further harm to both the individual struggling with addiction and the entire family unit. Recognising the signs that intervention is necessary is crucial in order to protect the emotional and physical wellbeing of everyone involved.

1. **Noticeable changes in behaviour, mood, or health:** Sudden or severe shifts in a family member's behaviour, such as mood swings, withdrawal, or physical health decline, can be signs that addiction is taking a toll. These changes often affect family dynamics, leading to confusion, stress, and concern among loved ones.

2. **Escalating conflicts or violence within the home:** As addiction deepens, it can fuel conflicts, arguments, and even violent behaviours. Tensions within the family may increase, with members feeling unsafe or emotionally drained. Intervention is essential when these dynamics become destructive.

3. **Financial instability linked to addictive habits:** Addiction often leads to financial strain, whether through over-spending, job loss, or mismanagement of resources. This instability can place immense pressure on the family, affecting the home environment and creating stress for all members, particularly children.

4. **Evidence of harm or neglect affecting children:** If addiction leads to neglect or harm towards children, it is imperative to act immediately. Signs include emotional or physical neglect, inconsistent caregiving, or children expressing fear, anxiety, or confusion about their home life.

Interventions can take many forms, from gentle conversations to seeking professional mediation. Regardless of the method, the goal is to restore balance and ensure the safety, stability, and wellbeing of the entire family, particularly children, while ensuring the safety and stability of the family.

Conclusion

The intersection of addiction and family life, especially when children are involved, is fraught with challenges, although not without hope. By understanding the complex interplay of these dynamics, families can work together to navigate the path to recovery. It requires courage, effort, and the willingness to face difficult truths; however, the rewards - restored relationships, stability, and wellbeing - are immeasurable. Let this chapter serve as a reminder that healing is possible, not just for the individual, it is possible for the entire family unit.

CHAPTER 29

THE CONNECTION BETWEEN ADDICTION AND LOSS

Loss, whether through bereavement, the end of a relationship, or any profound life change, is an inevitable part of the human experience. However, the way individuals respond to loss varies widely, shaped by personal resilience, coping mechanisms, and support systems. For some, the emotional pain of loss becomes overwhelming, and in their struggle to manage or escape it, they may turn to addictive behaviours or substances. This chapter explores the intricate relationship between addiction and loss, examining the psychological underpinnings, the reasons for this connection, and practical steps for healing and support.

The connection between loss and addiction

Loss is a profound and often life-altering experience, touching every corner of our emotional and mental being. Whether through bereavement, the end of a relationship, or other significant changes, it can leave us feeling untethered, vulnerable, and overwhelmed. In the midst of this emotional turmoil, some may turn to addictive behaviours or substances as a way to cope, numb the pain, or regain a sense of control. The connection between addiction and loss is deeply rooted in our psychological and neurological responses to grief. Understanding this link is essential for recognising the signs, addressing the underlying pain, and fostering a path toward healing and recovery.

Understanding the connection

At its core, addiction often serves as an attempt to fill a void, suppress emotional pain, or regain a sense of control. Loss disrupts an individual's sense of stability, creating a chasm where familiar routines, emotional anchors, and security once resided. In the face of this disruption:

1. **Emotional pain becomes intolerable:** Loss often triggers feelings of grief, despair, guilt, and anger. These emotions can feel unbearable, especially if the individual lacks healthy coping mechanisms. Substances like alcohol, drugs, or compulsive behaviours (e.g., gambling, overeating) may temporarily numb this pain.

2. **A need for escape:** People experiencing grief may feel trapped in their emotions or overwhelmed by the finality of their loss. Addiction offers a means of escape - albeit a fleeting and destructive one - from the reality they cannot yet face.

3. **A desire for control:** Bereavement often brings a sense of helplessness. Addiction, though harmful, may create an illusion of agency - something the person can 'control' (see Chapter 23) amidst the chaos of their emotions.

4. **Reinforcement of vulnerable pathways:** For individuals with a predisposition to addiction, either through genetics, past trauma, or prior substance use, loss can act as a trigger. The brain's reward system, already primed for addictive

behaviours, seizes on substances or actions that provide temporary relief.

Why it happens

The connection between addiction and loss is rooted in the psychological and neurological effects of grief:

1. **The brain's response to stress:** Loss activates the brain's stress response, releasing cortisol and other stress hormones. Chronic stress can impair the brain's ability to regulate emotions, increasing vulnerability to addictive behaviours as a means of self-soothing.

2. **The role of dopamine:** Substances and addictive behaviours stimulate the brain's release of dopamine, creating a sense of pleasure or relief. During grief, when natural dopamine levels may be suppressed, these artificial boosts become particularly enticing.

3. **Unprocessed grief:** In some cases, individuals may suppress or deny their grief, believing it is too painful to confront. Addiction often arises as a way to avoid the process of mourning; however, this avoidance exacerbates both the grief and the addiction over time.

4. **Social isolation:** Grieving individuals may withdraw from friends and family, either because they feel misunderstood or because they want to avoid burdening others. This isolation can compound feelings of loneliness, making certain substances or behaviours a substitute for human connection.

Steps to address addiction and loss

Recognising and addressing the link between addiction and loss requires a multi-faceted approach that combines self-awareness, professional help, and a supportive environment.

1. **Acknowledging the pain:** Healing begins with accepting the reality of loss. Suppressing or denying grief only deepens the emotional wounds. Journaling, speaking with trusted friends, or joining a bereavement group can help in processing feelings.

2. **Seeking professional support:** Therapists trained in grief counselling or addiction recovery can provide invaluable guidance. Cognitive behavioural therapy (CBT), trauma-focused therapy, or group support programmes like Alcoholics Anonymous (AA) can address both grief and addictive behaviours.

3. **Building healthy coping mechanisms:** Replacing harmful habits with constructive ones is crucial. Mindfulness, meditation, exercise, or creative outlets like art and music can provide relief from overwhelming emotions.

4. **Reconnecting with others:** Loss can leave people feeling isolated. Rebuilding social connections, whether through family, friends, or support groups, can offer a sense of belonging and reduce the temptation to seek solace in addiction.

5. **Understanding triggers:** Grieving individuals may find certain dates, places, or memories especially painful. Identifying these triggers and developing a plan to cope with them – such as creating new traditions or practising grounding techniques – can reduce the likelihood of relapse.

Chapter 29

When to seek help

Grief is a natural and deeply personal response to loss, although when addiction intertwines with the grieving process, it can hinder emotional healing and intensify the struggle. Recognising when to seek help is vital to regaining balance and addressing both grief and addictive behaviours. Professional support can provide the tools and guidance needed to navigate these complex emotions. Consider seeking help in the following scenarios:

1. **Substance use escalates:** If the use of alcohol, drugs, or other coping mechanisms begins to increase in frequency, intensity, or dependency, it's a clear sign that intervention is needed. This escalation may initially seem like a temporary way to manage pain; however, it can quickly evolve into a destructive pattern that deepens emotional distress and prolongs healing.

2. **Physical or emotional health declines:** Grief can manifest physically and emotionally, although persistent or worsening changes - such as rapid weight loss or gain, disrupted sleep patterns, chronic fatigue, or heightened emotional instability - indicate the need for professional support. These symptoms may signal that the combination of grief and addiction is overwhelming the body and mind.

3. **Social withdrawal increases:** Isolation is common during grief; however, if it becomes pervasive and leads to the severing of social ties, it can create a fertile ground for addictive behaviours. Isolation not only reinforces unhealthy habits; it also deprives the individual of the support and connection crucial for healing. Seeking help can rebuild these connections and foster a sense of belonging.

4. **Grief remains unresolved:** While grief has no fixed timeline, being stuck in an overwhelming cycle of sadness, anger, or numbness for months or even years can indicate the presence of complicated grief. This prolonged state can often co-occur with addiction, creating a vicious cycle that therapy can help break. Professionals trained in grief counselling can guide individuals toward resolution and recovery.

5. **Functionality becomes impaired:** If grief and addiction start to interfere with day-to-day responsibilities - such as work, relationships, or self-care - it's time to seek help. Struggling to maintain a routine or fulfil obligations is a strong indication that the burden has become too heavy to manage alone.

6. **Feelings of hopelessness or despair persist:** If grief feels unbearable and leads to persistent thoughts of hopelessness or despair, it's essential to reach out for help immediately. These feelings can be exacerbated by addiction and may require the intervention of mental health professionals to ensure safety and stability.

Grief is challenging, and when paired with addiction, it can hinder healing. Recognising when to seek help is key to breaking this cycle. With support, individuals can process grief, recover, and rebuild their lives, emerging stronger over time.

Conclusion

Though the link between addiction and loss can feel overwhelming, it is important to remember that healing is possible. The journey begins with small steps: recognising the pain, seeking help, and choosing healthier ways to cope. Over time, individuals can emerge from their grief not only with a greater understanding of their loss but also with a deeper resilience and capacity for growth.

Loss changes us; however, it does not have to define us. With the right support and resources, those affected by addiction and bereavement can rediscover hope and move forward with renewed purpose.

CHAPTER 30

THE CONNECTION BETWEEN ADDICTION AND WORK

Addiction and one's professional life are often interconnected in profound and complex ways. The interplay between workplace demands, personal vulnerabilities, and cultural influences can lead to, or exacerbate, addictive behaviours. This chapter explores the intricacies of this connection, shedding light on its causes, consequences, and solutions, as well as providing practical advice for individuals and organisations.

The connection between work and addiction

High-pressure work environments, long hours, and cultural norms within industries can drive individuals to rely on certain substances or behaviours as coping mechanisms. Whether it's alcohol, drugs, or workaholism itself, addiction can stem from the stress, isolation, or expectations tied to work. Understanding this relationship is crucial for recognising warning signs, addressing root causes, and creating healthier workplaces where success and wellbeing can coexist.

How addiction and work intertwine

Working can both enable and conceal addiction. The demands of modern workplaces often create an environment where addiction can thrive unnoticed for extended periods. Let's explore this relationship in more detail:

1. **Pressure to perform:** Industries such as finance, medicine, law, and technology often demand long hours, perfection, and quick decision-making. This relentless pressure can push professionals to seek substances or behaviours (e.g., excessive caffeine, alcohol, or even prescription stimulants) that help them stay alert or unwind. *Example:* A junior lawyer working 80-hour weeks may turn to prescription stimulants to meet deadlines, unaware of the long-term risks for health and dependency.

2. **Workplace social norms:** Many jobs encourage networking in settings where alcohol consumption is prevalent. For example, post-work drinks may start as a casual social habit and then gradually become a dependency, especially for individuals struggling with stress or anxiety. *Example:* In the advertising industry, frequent parties and client dinners can normalise heavy drinking, blurring the line between socialising and addiction.

3. **Roles that encourage isolation:** Jobs such as remote tech work, long-haul trucking, or freelancing can lead to loneliness and lack of supervision. This isolation can create opportunities for unmonitored addictive behaviours.

4. **Reward culture:** Professionals driven by high-stakes incentives often develop a cycle of 'work hard, reward harder'. Substance use, gambling, or binge behaviours may feel like justified rewards after intense work periods.

Chapter 30

Why there is a connection

The connection between addiction and work lies in the interaction of environmental triggers, individual psychology, and biological factors. Here's why this bond is so pervasive:

1. **Stress and cortisol:** Stress is a universal part of most jobs; however, chronic stress has significant physiological effects. Cortisol, the stress hormone, disrupts the brain's reward pathways, making it harder to experience pleasure from normal activities. Substances like alcohol or drugs artificially activate these pathways, creating a cycle of dependence.

2. **The search for escape:** Many professionals view their career as a means of providing security, status, and identity. However, when the career feels unfulfilling or overwhelming, they may turn to addiction as a way to escape these feelings. *Example:* A mid-career manager experiencing stagnation may find solace in binge-drinking or gambling, temporarily alleviating feelings of dissatisfaction.

3. **Culture of tolerance:** Some industries have a culture that tacitly accepts or even glamorises unhealthy habits. For example, Silicon Valley's 'hustle culture' may encourage the use of substances to stay productive, while the entertainment industry often normalises recreational drug use.

4. **Neurochemical cycles:** Addiction hijacks the brain's reward system, creating a craving for the same 'high' over and over. Similarly, achieving professional success - landing a big deal or receiving a promotion - can mirror this effect, leading some to chase that high through workaholism or other addictive behaviours.

How it happens

Addiction rarely develops in isolation. Several workplace and personal risk factors contribute to its emergence:

1. **High expectations and limited support:** In high-stress careers, employees may lack the resources or support to manage challenges healthily. Without outlets like therapy or mentoring, addiction can become a coping strategy.

2. **Workplace hierarchies:** Power dynamics may deter individuals from seeking help. For example, a junior employee might fear repercussions if they disclose their struggles.

3. **Perfectionism:** Individuals with perfectionist tendencies may push themselves to unhealthy limits. When they inevitably fall short of their self-imposed standards, substances or behaviours offer temporary relief.

4. **Accessibility of substances:** Certain industries provide easier access to addictive substances. For example, bartenders, chefs, or event planners may find themselves surrounded by alcohol, while others may have access to prescription medications.

5. **Shift work and fatigue:** Night shifts or irregular schedules can disrupt sleep and wellbeing, increasing reliance on substances like caffeine, alcohol, or drugs.

What to do about it

Breaking the cycle of addiction in a professional setting requires a combination of personal action, organisational reform, and societal change. Here are expanded strategies:

1. **For Individuals:**
   - **Self-reflection:** Begin by recognising patterns of behaviour. Are you using alcohol to relax every evening after work? Are you relying on stimulants to stay awake during long hours?
   - **Set boundaries:** Establish clear work-life boundaries to prevent burnout. Commit to activities that nourish your mental health, such as exercise, hobbies, or family time.
   - **Seek professional help:** Therapy can uncover underlying emotional or psychological issues driving addiction. For substance dependency, consider rehabilitation or support groups like Alcoholics Anonymous or SMART Recovery.

2. **For organisations:**
   - **Promote mental health resources:** Offer access to counselling services, stress management workshops, and flexible schedules.
   - **Re-evaluate workplace culture:** Create a culture that values wellbeing over relentless productivity. Discourage after-hours communication and foster open conversations about mental health.
   - **Train leaders:** Equip managers to recognise the signs of addiction and provide support without judgment.

3. **For society:**
   - **Challenge stigma:** Addiction should be seen as a health issue, not a moral failing. Public campaigns and education programmes can help normalise seeking help.
   - **Policy advocacy:** Governments can implement regulations to prevent exploitative work environments and fund accessible mental health services.

Building a path forward

Recovering from addiction requires patience and ongoing effort. It is not a linear process yet a journey involving setbacks and progress. Here are some practices to maintain long-term health:

1. **Create a support network:** Surround yourself with understanding colleagues, friends, and mentors who can help you stay accountable.

2. **Focus on holistic wellbeing:** Incorporate mindfulness, nutrition, and physical activity into your routine to build resilience.

3. **Celebrate small wins:** Acknowledge progress, no matter how minor. This reinforces motivation and strengthens your commitment to recovery.

When to seek help

In the workplace, addiction can often go unnoticed until it has significantly impacted performance, relationships, and overall wellbeing. However, early intervention is key in preventing addiction from escalating into a more serious issue. Recognising when it's time to seek help - whether for yourself or a colleague - can make all the difference in ensuring long-term recovery and maintaining a healthy work-life balance. Below are critical moments when it's essential to act and seek support in a career context.

1. **At the first warning signs:** Recognising early signs of addiction in the workplace is vital to prevent escalation and support recovery. Indicators include frequent absenteeism, declining performance, mood swings, and noticeable physical changes like fatigue or neglecting appearance. Addressing these signs promptly ensures timely intervention, helping individuals regain control of their health and work life.

2. **After a significant stressor:** High-stress work events can trigger addiction as individuals turn to unhealthy coping mechanisms. Recognising these moments and addressing addiction early can prevent long-term dependency and help individuals develop healthier ways to manage stress.

3. **If others express concern:** Addiction is often hard for individuals to recognise early; however, colleagues, managers, or family members may notice behavioural changes first. Taking their concerns seriously and offering support can prevent escalation, helping the individual realise they need help before the issue worsens.

Addiction in the workplace can impact an individual's career, health, and relationships. Recognising when to seek help – whether at the first signs, after a stressor, or when others express concern – is crucial for preventing escalation. Early intervention provides support and helps individuals regain control, maintain success, and thrive both professionally and personally.

My personal experience

I have always enjoyed what I do for a living. It has given me so many wonderful experiences and opportunities. Work gives me structure, identity, pride, and purpose. However, it also became my escape. It was where I went to avoid feelings, to stay busy enough not to notice I wasn't okay. I could stay busy 24 hours a day, seven days a week. Over time, work became my fixation. Learning to set boundaries, and to find worth beyond productivity, was a turning point in me resetting my focus. I still work just as hard as I have

> ever worked, only now I take some time for myself, as well as doing as much as I can for others.

Conclusion

The connection between addiction and work is shaped by the pressures, expectations, and culture of the workplace. By understanding its causes and recognising its signs, individuals and organisations can address this issue proactively. A fulfilling career and a healthy life are not mutually exclusive; with the right strategies, it is possible to thrive in both arenas while maintaining balance and wellbeing.

CHAPTER 31

THE CONNECTION BETWEEN ADDICTION AND HIGH ACHIEVERS

At first glance, addiction and high achievement may seem worlds apart. One suggests dysfunction, dependency, and self-destruction; the other conjures images of discipline, success, and resilience. Yet, beneath the surface, the two often intersect in powerful, complex, and surprising ways. This chapter explores the psychological, neurological, and environmental links between addiction and high achievement, and offers guidance on how to recognise, understand, and manage this connection.

The connection between high achievers and addiction

The link between high achievement and addiction is not coincidental – it's systemic. Modern society rewards output, excellence, and image. There is little space for vulnerability, and emotional needs are frequently subordinated to goals. In such an environment, high achievers are praised for pushing boundaries, often without regard to the cost to their health.

Moreover, addiction is not simply about substances – it's about compulsion, escapism, and control (see Chapter 6). High achievers often strive for control in their professional lives, and addiction can represent either an extension of this control (e.g., using substances/behaviours to improve performance) or a rebellion against it (e.g., using to escape the pressure).

In some cases, addiction arises not in spite of success, but because of it. The higher one climbs, the more isolated, pressured, and scrutinised one can feel. Addiction can emerge as a form of self-medication or emotional levelling.

The psychology behind the connection

High achievers are often driven by intense internal motivations and deep psychological dynamics. While these traits can fuel extraordinary success, they also make individuals vulnerable to addiction. Understanding the psychological and neurobiological factors that link high achievement and addiction helps to shed light on why addiction is so common - yet often hidden - in high achievers.

1. **Perfectionism and high self-expectations:** High achievers frequently set impossibly high standards for themselves, creating chronic stress and fear of failure that addiction can temporarily numb.

2. **Emotional suppression and avoidance:** To maintain their 'on' persona, many suppress difficult emotions. Addiction offers a false refuge from feelings that seem unsafe or overwhelming.

3. **Reward system sensitivity:** The brain's reward pathways can become overly reliant on substances or behaviours that trigger dopamine surges, reinforcing addictive patterns.

4. **Cognitive distortions:** Black-and-white thinking, catastrophising, and overgeneralisation are common in high

achievers, intensifying feelings of inadequacy and driving compulsive behaviour.

5. **Imposter syndrome and self-doubt:** Despite outward success, many high achievers struggle with internal doubts about their worth, leading to self-medicating or escape through addiction.

6. **Early life experiences:** Childhood environments that emphasised achievement over emotional expression can predispose individuals to addictive coping styles later in life.

How are high achievers vulnerable to addiction?

High achievers are often lauded for their drive, ambition, and relentless pursuit of goals. However, these very traits can also predispose individuals to addictive behaviours. Several key factors contribute to this paradox:

1. **Perfectionism and pressure:** High achievers frequently operate under immense pressure - often self-imposed - to perform, succeed, and exceed expectations. This can create a mental environment where any perceived failure is intolerable. Substances or addictive behaviours can offer momentary relief from this unrelenting inner critic.

2. **High dopamine sensitivity:** Many high achievers have high-functioning brains that crave stimulation. Their neurological reward systems may be more sensitive to dopamine - the 'pleasure chemical' involved in both reward and addiction. This makes them more susceptible to the quick hits of satisfaction that addictive substances or behaviours provide.

3. **All-or-nothing thinking:** The same mindset that drives

excellence - intensity, focus, and an all-in attitude - can also foster extremes. Whether it's work, fitness, gambling, or alcohol, high achievers often go full tilt. This personality type can struggle with moderation, making addiction a greater risk.

4. **Burnout and emotional suppression:** Success often comes at the cost of emotional neglect. In prioritising goals, high achievers may ignore or suppress emotional needs, only for these to manifest through unhealthy coping mechanisms later on.

How addiction happens to high achievers

The journey from high performance to dependency is rarely a dramatic fall - more often it's a slow erosion. It might start innocuously: a glass of wine after work to 'unwind,' the use of stimulants to meet deadlines, or endless scrolling as a mental escape. Gradually, these behaviours become regular, then necessary, then habitual. This shift can be particularly hard to spot due to the ability to maintain external success while concealing internal struggles. Here's how addiction typically develops in high achievers:

1. **Initial coping mechanism:** It often starts with an occasional behaviour used to manage stress or enhance performance - a glass of wine to unwind, a stimulant to stay focused, or compulsive digital use to escape mentally. These actions are socially acceptable and may even be encouraged in high-performance environments.

2. **Positive reinforcement:** The behaviour 'works' - at least temporarily. It reduces anxiety, improves concentration, or helps disconnect. The brain registers this as a reward, and the action is repeated.

3. **Increased frequency and emotional reliance:** Over time, the behaviour becomes more frequent. It is no longer just a tool for occasional stress relief - it starts to feel necessary to function. Emotional regulation becomes increasingly tied to the behaviour or substance.

4. **Integration into routine:** The behaviour becomes part of daily life. It may be scheduled - the evening drink, the morning pill, the late-night scrolling. Attempts to cut back or reduce bring discomfort. It starts to feel automatic, almost non-negotiable.

5. **Justification and rationalisation:** High achievers often justify these behaviours: 'I deserve it after a long day,' or 'It helps me perform better.' Because they continue to succeed externally, they see little reason to question or stop.

6. **Masking and high-functioning addiction:** Despite the growing reliance, the individual continues to achieve, out-perform, and meet expectations. To outsiders - and often to high achievers themselves - there appears to be no problem. This is known as 'high-functioning addiction' and is especially dangerous because it hides in plain sight.

7. **Resistance to vulnerability or help:** Traits that drive success - independence, control, and perfectionism - become obstacles. Admitting to a problem feels like failure. Seeking help is seen as weakness. The cycle continues, unchallenged. Until it doesn't.

8. **Breaking point or collapse:** Eventually, the cost becomes unavoidable - whether through burnout, a health crisis, relationship issues, or emotional breakdown. This often becomes the turning point where the issue can no longer be ignored.

Reimagining success: a new model for achievement

For many high achievers, the traditional definition of success - focused on status, speed, and constant growth - can become a trap rather than a goal. This narrow view often drives relentless effort, emotional suppression, and ultimately burnout or addiction. It creates pressure to keep pushing forward, even at the cost of personal wellbeing and authentic happiness.

Redefining success is not about abandoning ambition or lowering standards. Instead, it means reshaping how we understand achievement so that it supports both excellence and holistic wellbeing. By embracing a broader, more sustainable vision of success, high achievers can break free from harmful cycles and cultivate a life that is fulfilling, balanced, and resilient.

Here is a more balanced model of success, centred on six key principles:

1. **Emotional awareness and balance:** Develop the ability to recognise and manage emotions. Emotional self-awareness supports better decision-making, reduces stress, and builds resilience.

2. **Authentic relationships:** Foster connections that are honest and supportive. Meaningful relationships remind you that your value extends beyond your achievements.

3. **Rest and renewal:** Prioritise rest, leisure, and joyful experiences. These are not distractions; they are essential components of sustainable high performance.

4. **Purpose-driven ambition:** Align your goals with your values. When your efforts serve a deeper purpose, they become more fulfilling and less dependent on external validation.

5. **Healthy boundaries and self-respect:** Protect your energy and mental space by setting clear limits with work, technology, and others. Boundaries allow room for growth without collapse.

6. **Self-defined success:** Measure progress by your own standards. Replace the need for constant external approval with internal satisfaction and long-term vision.

This updated approach allows high achievers to remain ambitious while also being whole, well, and grounded. It encourages a kind of success that can be lived - not just performed.

When to seek help

Understanding the connection between addiction and high achievement is only the first step; knowing how to respond is equally vital. This section outlines practical steps to take, when to take them, and how to shift from reactive coping to proactive care - without sacrificing ambition or success.

1. **Recognise the signs early:** Early intervention is key. Look for patterns of dependency - not just in substances, also in behaviours: workaholism, compulsive exercising, perfectionism, or digital overuse. Recognise when a coping mechanism becomes a necessity.

2. **Challenge the 'success at all costs' mindset:** Redefine success to include wellbeing, rest, and emotional health. High achievement must be sustainable. If success requires the sacrifice of health or sanity, it is, ultimately, self-defeating.

3. **Create safe spaces for vulnerability:** High achievers often struggle to ask for help. Promote environments - in workplaces, families, and social groups - where emotional

honesty is not only permitted; it is encouraged.

4. **Professional support is not a weakness:** Encourage therapy, coaching, or counselling as routine components of a healthy, high-functioning life. Just as a high performer sees a personal trainer, they should feel no stigma in consulting a therapist.

5. **Rebalance the reward system:** Addiction hijacks the brain's reward system. Reintroduce healthy sources of dopamine: physical activity, creativity, nature, meaningful relationships. Mindfulness practices can also help rewire the brain for healthier satisfaction.

6. **Know the triggers and timing:** Major transitions - promotions, burnout, retirement, or personal crises - are peak moments for vulnerability. Anticipate these changes and proactively engage support systems during these periods.

Conclusion

The connection between addiction and high achievement is not a contradiction - it is a reflection of human complexity. The same traits that fuel greatness can, when unbalanced, drive self-destruction. However, understanding this link offers hope and a starting point. By integrating emotional intelligence, balance, and mental health into the concept of success, high achievers can not only reach their goals; they can also live a life of depth, connection, and wholeness.

CHAPTER 32

THE CONNECTION BETWEEN ADDICTION AND OVERWORKING

In an era that glorifies productivity and hustle, overworking has evolved into a modern-day addiction. This phenomenon is not limited to those striving for success, it touches many, from corporate professionals to entrepreneurs, academics, and even caregivers. Although addiction is most commonly associated with substances such as drugs or alcohol, overworking shares a similarly compulsive nature that traps people in a cycle of dependency, often to the detriment of their health, relationships, and overall wellbeing.

The connection between overworking and addiction

In today's fast-paced, success-driven world, the line between dedication and overworking often blurs, leading to a troubling overlap between addiction and excessive work habits. While addiction is typically associated with substances or behaviours like gambling, overworking exhibits many of the same compulsive patterns.

The nature of addiction and overworking

Addiction is fundamentally a psychological and physiological dependence on a substance or behaviour. At its core, addiction involves repeated engagement with a particular activity despite adverse consequences. In the case of overworking, the addictive element lies in the rush of achievement and the sense of purpose that relentless work can provide. However, just like substance abuse, overworking can ultimately spiral into an unmanageable problem, leading to exhaustion, burnout, and even severe health issues, such as heart disease, depression, and anxiety.

Addiction to overworking is often referred to as 'workaholism.' While it may not manifest in the same visible ways as traditional addiction, the underlying dynamics are startlingly similar. Workaholics derive a sense of identity and validation from their productivity, becoming reliant on the act of working to fulfil emotional needs. Much like other addictions, this behaviour often escalates, requiring more and more work to maintain the same psychological satisfaction.

Why it happens

The connection between addiction and overworking is multifaceted, rooted in a combination of societal pressures, psychological vulnerabilities, and neurological factors.

1. **Societal expectations:** Modern culture frequently celebrates overworking, equating it with ambition, dedication, and success. Phrases like 'hustle culture' and 'grind' have become mantras in professional spheres, encouraging people to glorify busyness. This social endorsement makes it difficult to recognise overworking as problematic because, in many circles, it is seen as admirable rather than harmful.

2. **Psychological factors:** People with underlying psychological predispositions, such as perfectionism, low self-esteem, or a need for control, are more vulnerable to developing an

addiction to work. Overworking allows them to distract from uncomfortable emotions, such as anxiety or inadequacy, while also giving them a sense of mastery and achievement.

3. **Neurological mechanisms:** Overworking triggers the brain's reward system, releasing dopamine - the neurotransmitter we've talked about throughout this book that is associated with pleasure and motivation. Over time, the brain becomes conditioned to seek out this reward, reinforcing the behaviour and making it difficult to disengage from work. Similar to other forms of addiction, the brain begins to crave more work to release the same amount of dopamine, resulting in a never-ending cycle.

How overworking becomes an addiction

The transformation from normal work habits into an addiction is often gradual, making it difficult to pinpoint when things take a turn for the worse. Many overworkers initially begin by taking on extra tasks to meet a deadline or prove their worth; however, over time, this becomes a default mode of operation. As the person takes on more and more work, they begin to experience diminishing returns - yet they feel an increasing compulsion to continue.

This pattern becomes an addiction when the person can no longer control their engagement with work. They may continue working beyond their capacity, ignoring signs of physical and mental distress, such as fatigue, insomnia, or irritability. Just as a person addicted to a substance experiences withdrawal symptoms when not using, a workaholic may feel anxious, restless, or even depressed during periods of inactivity.

The psychological drivers of work addiction

Several psychological mechanisms can drive overworking, turning it from a productive habit into a destructive addiction:

1. **Validation and self-worth:** Many people derive their sense of self-worth from external achievements. In such cases, work becomes the primary way to gain approval and validation from others, whether through praise, promotions, or financial rewards. Over time, their identity becomes entwined with their professional accomplishments, making it difficult to separate who they are from what they do.

2. **Escapism:** Overworking often serves as a form of escapism, providing a distraction from emotional difficulties or unresolved personal issues. Those facing relationship problems, grief, or anxiety may bury themselves in work to avoid confronting painful emotions. The temporary relief provided by focusing on tasks and deadlines can create a dependency on work as a coping mechanism.

3. **Control:** In a world filled with uncertainties, work offers a sense of control. Being busy allows people to feel that they are managing their environment effectively, even if other areas of their life are out of balance. This need for control can fuel overworking tendencies, as individuals seek to micromanage every aspect of their professional responsibilities.

The consequences of overworking addiction

While overworking might seem like a productive vice, the consequences are significant and far-reaching. Physically, overworking can lead to chronic stress, heart problems, and a weakened immune system. Mentally, it can result in burnout, depression, and anxiety.

Socially, workaholism isolates individuals from friends, family, and loved ones, as they prioritise their work over personal relationships.

The costs are not merely personal; it can also impact the organisation and community. Overworked employees may initially appear more productive; however, they are more likely to experience burnout, make mistakes, and show reduced creativity in the long term. Workaholism also encourages toxic work cultures where long hours are expected, pressuring others to overwork as well.

Recognising and addressing work addiction

Recognising work addiction is often the first step towards addressing the issue. Individuals need to reflect on their relationship with work and ask themselves difficult questions:

- Do I feel anxious or guilty when I'm not working?
- Have I sacrificed my health, relationships, or personal happiness for the sake of work?
- Am I using work to avoid dealing with personal issues or emotions?

If the answer to these questions is yes, it may be time to reassess your work habits.

What to do

Addressing work addiction involves practical steps and strategies. This section offers actionable recommendations to help individuals regain balance and fulfilment.

1. **Set boundaries:** One of the most effective ways to combat work addiction is by setting clear boundaries around work. Establishing set working hours and taking regular breaks is crucial. Time away from work should be used to recharge mentally

and physically, whether through hobbies, social interactions, or relaxation.

2. **Delegate and say no:** Many workaholics struggle with the idea of delegation, fearing that others won't meet their standards. However, learning to delegate and say no to unnecessary tasks is essential for breaking the cycle of overworking. It requires trusting others to take responsibility and acknowledging that perfection is neither possible nor necessary.

3. **Address underlying issues:** Overworking is often a symptom of deeper psychological issues. Speaking to a counsellor or therapist can help individuals uncover and address these underlying factors. Cognitive behavioural therapy (CBT) and mindfulness techniques can be particularly helpful in shifting unhealthy thought patterns around work and control.

4. **Re-evaluate success:** Redefining what success looks like is key. Rather than equating success solely with professional achievement, individuals should explore other dimensions of fulfilment, such as personal growth, relationships, and well-being. A more holistic view of success encourages a healthier balance between work and life.

5. **Take time off:** Regular holidays and time away from work can help reset unhealthy patterns. It's important to fully disconnect during these periods, avoiding the temptation to check emails or take calls. Time away allows the mind and body to recover, which ultimately leads to greater productivity in the long run.

When to seek help

If overworking has begun to severely impact your health, relationships, or overall quality of life, it may be time to seek professional help. Ignoring the signs of work addiction can lead to chronic burnout, mental health issues, and strained personal connections. The sooner workaholism is recognised and addressed, the easier it is to prevent further damage. Early intervention can help you break the cycle of overworking and regain control over your wellbeing.

1. **Persistent physical symptoms:** If you're experiencing ongoing fatigue, frequent illness, or chronic headaches that don't seem to improve with rest, it could be a sign that your body is overwhelmed by the demands of work. These physical symptoms can indicate that overworking is affecting your health, and professional help can provide the support needed to recover.

2. **Mental health struggles:** Overworking can contribute to anxiety, depression, and/or stress that interferes with your daily life. If you're feeling overwhelmed, mentally drained, or unable to focus on anything other than work, it may be time to speak to a therapist or counsellor who can help you address the emotional toll of excessive working.

3. **Relationship strain:** If your work is causing distance between you and your loved ones, colleagues, or friends, it's a sign that the balance is tipped too far towards work. Constantly prioritising work over personal connections can damage relationships. Therapy or coaching can help you learn how to set boundaries and restore your relationships.

4. **Inability to disconnect:** If you find it impossible to stop thinking about work during your downtime, or feel guilty about taking breaks, you may be dealing with work addiction. A coach or therapist can help you develop strategies to disconnect from work and focus on recovery.

5. **Lack of self-care:** If you are neglecting self-care activities such as eating well, exercising, or sleeping because of work, it's

essential to reassess your priorities. Professional help can assist you in creating healthier routines that prioritise both work and personal wellbeing.

6. **Escalating stress levels:** When work-induced stress begins to feel unmanageable, and no amount of time off or rest helps, seeking professional guidance is critical. A mental health professional can help you cope with stress and find better ways to manage your workload.

7. **Burnout symptoms:** If you're experiencing burnout - feeling emotionally exhausted, detached, or ineffective in your work (see Chapter 33) - professional assistance can help you understand the root causes and offer ways to recover. Support groups, coaching, or therapy can provide the tools needed to heal from burnout and prevent future episodes.

The sooner workaholism is identified and addressed, the easier it is to manage. Early intervention can prevent the cycle of overworking from causing more severe damage, both mentally and physically.

My personal experience

I didn't just work hard - I overworked to exhaustion. I love being busy! I love what I do - the connection, the purpose. Working with people, connecting, guiding, building, developing... it is a privilege. Overworking gave me a sense of purpose. However, it came at the cost of my health, my presence with family, and my peace of mind. If you keep going at 100 mph and don't slow down at any point over a long distance, it is only a matter of time before something goes wrong or you become overwhelmed. Slowing down wasn't just necessary – it was lifesaving. It gave me peace of mind and internal comfort. Not to mention precious time, spent in the present, with my family.

Conclusion

The connection between addiction and overworking is not always obvious, yet it is prevalent in modern society. While hard work is often celebrated and rewarded, the compulsive nature of work addiction can lead to burnout, physical illness, and personal dissatisfaction. Recognising the signs and taking action to break the cycle are critical to maintaining a healthy and balanced life.

By re-evaluating priorities, setting boundaries, and addressing the psychological roots of overworking, individuals can break free from this damaging pattern and rediscover joy in both their professional and personal lives.

CHAPTER 33

THE CONNECTION BETWEEN ADDICTION AND BURNOUT

Burnout and addiction are often treated as separate entities, yet they share significant underlying connections. Both conditions are responses to chronic stress and emotional exhaustion, while burnout typically results from prolonged exposure to overwhelming demands, addiction emerges as a coping mechanism, often to escape or numb the very feelings burnout brings. Understanding how these two phenomena intersect is crucial for addressing the root causes and creating effective strategies for recovery.

The connection between burnout and addiction

Burnout often creates a fertile ground for addiction to develop. When the body and mind are depleted, individuals may seek ways to temporarily alleviate their suffering. Substance abuse, whether it's alcohol, drugs, or prescription medication, becomes a form of self-medication to manage the emotional and physical toll burnout takes.

Similarly, behavioural addictions, such as compulsive gaming, gambling, or even workaholism, can emerge as a way to escape the uncomfortable feelings associated with burnout. These coping mechanisms provide a temporary distraction or relief, although it inevitably deepens the cycle of stress and exhaustion. Over time, addiction exacerbates burnout, creating a vicious cycle that becomes increasingly difficult to break.

Understanding burnout

Burnout is a state of physical, emotional, and mental exhaustion caused by long-term involvement in demanding situations. It is most commonly discussed in the context of work, although it can occur in any area of life where excessive stress is present - whether it's caring for a loved one, managing chronic health issues, or maintaining a high level of performance in any demanding role. Common symptoms of burnout include:

- Chronic fatigue, even after rest.
- Detachment from responsibilities and a sense of cynicism or negativity.
- Decreased productivity and feelings of ineffectiveness.
- Difficulty concentrating or making decisions.
- Physical symptoms like headaches, insomnia, or digestive problems.

Burnout is not simply stress; it is the prolonged inability to cope with the ongoing pressures of life, leaving the individual feeling empty and lacking motivation.

How it happens

Understanding the connection between burnout and addiction is crucial for recognising how these conditions reinforce each other. By exploring the psychological, neurological, and social factors involved, we can better comprehend why individuals may turn to addictive behaviours to cope with the toll of burnout.

1. **Emotional numbing:** Burnout leads to emotional exhaustion, and addictive substances or behaviours can numb those feelings. The temporary relief from stress and emotional pain becomes highly reinforcing, leading the person to repeatedly engage in the addictive behaviour.

2. **Dopamine deficit:** Burnout is associated with a decrease in dopamine, the neurotransmitter that regulates pleasure and reward. When someone is 'burnt out,' everyday activities no longer bring the satisfaction they once did. Addiction provides a shortcut to instant dopamine release, which can feel like the only way to experience pleasure or relief.

3. **Cognitive impairment:** Chronic stress impairs decision-making and impulse control, making it harder for individuals to resist engaging in addictive behaviours. The ability to reason and evaluate long-term consequences is diminished, increasing susceptibility to addiction.

4. **Isolation and disconnection:** Burnout often leads to withdrawal from social interactions, which can increase feelings of loneliness and despair. Addiction thrives in isolation, as individuals turn inward, retreating from the very support systems that might otherwise help them manage stress.

What to do

Recovery from burnout and addiction involves addressing both the emotional exhaustion and the unhealthy coping mechanisms that developed. It is not enough to tackle one without the other, as both conditions fuel each other.

1. **Acknowledge the burnout:** The first step is recognising burnout for what it is – a state of overwhelming stress that requires

immediate attention. This involves acknowledging that the body and mind need rest and that continuing at the current pace is unsustainable.

2. **Reassess priorities:** Often, burnout is the result of overcommitment. Take time to evaluate which aspects of your life or work are draining the most energy and whether they can be modified or eliminated. Learning to set boundaries and say no are both crucial.
3. **Develop healthy coping mechanisms:** Addiction often develops because people don't have effective ways of managing stress. Learning new skills, such as mindfulness, meditation, and relaxation techniques, can provide healthier ways to deal with emotional and physical exhaustion.
4. **Seek professional help:** Both burnout and addiction require professional intervention in many cases. Therapists, addiction specialists, and coaches can provide personalised guidance to address the root causes and develop a sustainable recovery plan.
5. **Build a support network:** Burnout and addiction both thrive in isolation. Rebuilding relationships and creating a support system of family, friends, or peers who understand what you're going through can help provide the emotional support needed during recovery.
6. **Pace yourself:** Recovery from burnout and addiction is not a quick fix. It's essential to take time for self-care and to avoid overloading yourself during the healing process. Gradually reintroduce responsibilities and activities to avoid falling back into the patterns that led to burnout.

Why addressing burnout helps prevent addiction

By addressing burnout before it spirals into addiction, individuals can reclaim their emotional and mental wellbeing. Tackling the root cause - chronic stress - can prevent the need for unhealthy coping mechanisms in the first place. Regular self-care, stress management, and boundary-setting are not just optional; they are essential to long-term health and happiness.

Understanding the connection between burnout and addiction can also help reduce the stigma associated with both. Too often, addiction is seen as a moral failing, when in reality, it is a response to overwhelming stress and emotional fatigue. By treating burnout, we can take proactive steps towards preventing addiction from taking root.

When to seek help

One of the critical factors in addressing the connection between burnout and addiction is recognising the signs early. The earlier intervention occurs, the better the chance of breaking the cycle. Here are some key moments when action is necessary:

1. **During the warning signs of burnout:** If you notice persistent signs of burnout - exhaustion, negativity, and/or reduced performance - this is the time to reassess your stress levels and workload. Seek support, whether from a counsellor, a trusted friend, or a healthcare provider, before turning to addictive substances or behaviours for relief.

2. **Before burnout deepens into addiction:** Once unhealthy coping mechanisms begin, such as relying on alcohol or drugs to unwind, it's crucial to acknowledge the problem. This is when prevention and intervention can halt addiction before it takes

root. Developing healthier coping strategies, such as mindfulness, exercise, or talking therapy, can make a huge difference.

3. **After recognising dependency:** If addiction has already developed, recognising this is not the end; it is rather the start of recovery. Seeking professional help through rehabilitation, counselling, or support groups can provide the necessary tools to break the addiction while addressing the burnout that led to it.

4. **Recognising burnout's impact on relationships:** Burnout not only affects the individual; it can also strain personal and professional relationships. If you notice your interactions with others becoming increasingly negative or withdrawn, this is an important moment to seek help. Addressing burnout early can help prevent it from affecting your social and professional life, potentially preventing a deeper reliance on addictive behaviours to cope with relational stress.

5. **Monitoring emotional and physical health:** Burnout often manifests through both physical and emotional symptoms. If there are signs such as chronic illness, insomnia, or emotional numbness, it's vital to seek help before these issues escalate. These physical and emotional indicators can lead to a reliance on substances to temporarily ease discomfort, and addressing them promptly can prevent addiction.

6. **Taking preventive action during high-risk situations:** Certain environments or periods in life, such as high-pressure jobs, caring for a loved one with illness, or undergoing significant life transitions, can increase the likelihood of burnout. Recognising these high-risk periods and taking proactive steps, such as seeking stress management resources or building a support system, can prevent both burnout and addiction.

Recognising burnout early and taking action before it leads to addiction is crucial. Addressing exhaustion, seeking support, and adopting healthier coping strategies can break the cycle. Early intervention helps protect wellbeing and relationships, and promotes lasting recovery.

My personal experience

Burnout didn't hit all at once for me. It was a slow erosion – of energy, joy, connection. I remember that it had started quite some time before I felt as if action was needed, a year or so. The constant drive, the need to push forward and succeed was relentless. I was relentless. By the time I got to Rainford Hall, I was running on fumes. I had lost who I was. I had completely run out of energy. Recovery started with recognising that burnout wasn't weakness – it was a signal. A message that something had to change.

Conclusion

The link between burnout and addiction is profound, and addressing this connection can be life changing. Burnout is an early warning sign that should never be ignored, as it can quickly lead to unhealthy behaviours that only deepen emotional and physical distress. By recognising the signs, seeking support, and developing healthier coping mechanisms, it is possible to break free from the cycle of burnout and addiction, leading to a healthier and more balanced life.

CHAPTER 34

THE CONNECTION BETWEEN ADDICTION AND BOREDOM

Addiction and boredom may appear to be unrelated phenomena at first glance; however, a closer examination reveals an intricate and significant connection between the two. Understanding this link is crucial for comprehending the complexities of addiction and developing effective strategies for prevention and intervention. This chapter delves into how boredom can contribute to the development and maintenance of addictive behaviours, why this connection exists, and what can be done to address it.

The connection between boredom and addiction

The connection between addiction and boredom lies in the way both shape human behaviour. Boredom often creates a sense of emptiness or dissatisfaction, leading individuals to seek out stimulation or relief, which can manifest in addictive behaviours. Whether through substances, gambling, or digital media, the temporary escape from boredom can reinforce unhealthy habits, making it difficult to break free. Understanding this link is crucial for addressing the root causes of addiction and developing strategies for healthier coping mechanisms.

Understanding the connection

Boredom can lead people to seek out addictive behaviours as a way to escape feelings of restlessness. By examining how boredom impacts the brain and behaviour, we can better understand the link between these two phenomena.

1. **How boredom fuels addiction:** Boredom, at its core, is a state of dissatisfaction and restlessness that arises when individuals feel they lack meaningful engagement or stimulation. This emotional state often drives people to seek out novel experiences, distractions, or pleasures. In the context of addiction, boredom can be a powerful catalyst, pushing individuals towards behaviours or substances that offer temporary relief from their ennui. Addictive behaviours often provide an escape from the monotony of everyday life. Whether it's substance abuse, gambling, or excessive use of digital media, these activities can offer an immediate sense of excitement, engagement, or reward. For someone feeling bored, these experiences can seem particularly alluring as they promise a break from the dullness of their routine.

2. **Why the connection exists:** The connection between boredom and addiction is rooted in several psychological and neurological factors. Firstly, boredom is associated with a need for stimulation and a sense of purpose. When individuals are unable to fulfil these needs through conventional means, they may turn to addictive behaviours as a way to satisfy them. Neurologically, boredom can affect the brain's reward system. When engaged in stimulating activities, the brain releases dopamine, a neurotransmitter associated with pleasure and reward. Boredom can diminish this dopamine release, leading individuals to seek out activities that artificially increase dopamine levels. Addictive substances and behaviours can hijack

this system, providing an exaggerated and temporary sense of pleasure that contrasts starkly with the feelings of boredom.

What makes the connection strong

The relationship between boredom and addiction is intensified by certain emotional and social factors. Emotional regulation difficulties, along with the overstimulation of modern society, make the temptation of addictive behaviours stronger when boredom strikes.

1. **The role of emotional regulation:** Addiction often involves difficulties with emotional regulation. Individuals who struggle with managing their emotions may find themselves more susceptible to addiction when faced with boredom. The feelings of emptiness and dissatisfaction associated with boredom can amplify emotional distress, leading individuals to seek solace in addictive behaviours.

2. **The impact of modern society:** In contemporary society, where constant stimulation is readily available through technology and media, the experience of boredom has become less frequent but more intense when it does occur. The rapid pace of modern life can make periods of boredom feel particularly stark and uncomfortable, exacerbating the desire to engage in addictive behaviours as a means of escaping these feelings.

What to do

Addressing boredom and its link to addiction requires adopting healthier coping strategies and creating environments that foster engagement. Recognising boredom as a trigger for addiction is the first step in breaking the cycle.

1. **Developing healthy coping strategies:** Addressing the

connection between boredom and addiction requires the development of healthy coping mechanisms. Individuals can benefit from learning new skills or engaging in activities that provide genuine satisfaction and fulfilment. This might include pursuing hobbies, setting personal goals, and/or participating in activities that foster a sense of purpose and achievement.

2. **Creating engaging environments:** For those in positions to influence others, such as educators, employers, or policymakers, creating environments that reduce boredom can be an effective strategy. This might involve offering opportunities for meaningful engagement, providing variety in daily routines, and encouraging activities that stimulate creativity and personal growth.

3. **Seeking professional support:** For individuals struggling with addiction, professional support is often essential. Therapists and counsellors can help individuals understand the underlying causes of their addiction, including boredom, and work with them to develop healthier coping strategies. Therapeutic approaches might include cognitive behavioural therapy (CBT), which can assist individuals in recognising and changing patterns of thinking and behaviour related to boredom and addiction.

When to seek help

Boredom can be a powerful trigger for addictive behaviours, and while occasional boredom is a natural part of life, persistent or overwhelming boredom may require attention. Recognising when boredom is leading to harmful coping mechanisms is crucial for addressing the underlying issues and preventing further harm. If boredom is causing distress or driving unhealthy habits, seeking help can provide valuable support and direction.

1. **Persistent feelings of emptiness:** If boredom continues over an extended period, leading to persistent feelings of emptiness or dissatisfaction, it may signal a need for professional support. Chronic boredom can sometimes mask deeper emotional or psychological issues that need to be addressed.

2. **Turning to addictive behaviours:** When boredom drives someone to repeatedly seek out substances, activities, or behaviours (like gambling or excessive screen time) to fill the void, it's time to consider help. These behaviours may temporarily alleviate boredom although they often lead to negative consequences.

3. **Difficulty finding meaning or purpose:** If boredom is accompanied by a sense of hopelessness or an inability to find meaning in daily activities, this can contribute to a deeper sense of despair. Professional guidance can help individuals explore underlying issues and find healthy ways to engage with life.

4. **Struggling with emotional regulation:** People who struggle to manage their emotions during periods of boredom may develop unhealthy coping strategies, such as substance abuse or compulsive behaviours. Therapy can assist in improving emotional regulation and finding healthier outlets.

5. **Escalating negative impact on daily life:** If boredom is interfering with work, relationships, or overall wellbeing, it's important to seek help. Addiction-related boredom often worsens over time, impacting various aspects of life, and addressing it early can prevent further harm.

By recognising these signs, individuals can take proactive steps to manage boredom healthily and prevent the cycle of addiction from taking hold. Seeking support from professionals can provide crucial tools for developing healthier ways to cope and find fulfilment.

My personal experience

At times, boredom would lead me to seek distractions that drained my energy rather than restored it. This included working more and working later. It wasn't until I began my reset that I recognised boredom as a trigger for me. Instead of seeing it as something negative, I started to view boredom as an opportunity to explore new experiences, interests or ideas, and develop healthier coping strategies. The restlessness I felt was often a signal that I needed to reconnect with meaningful activities and inner calm. It is a constant balance between keeping yourself busy from boredom and doing too much. Learning to sit with boredom without acting on the need to do something became a positive tool for healing and awareness.

Conclusion

The connection between boredom and addiction is a multifaceted issue that involves psychological, neurological, and societal factors. By understanding this connection, individuals and professionals can better address the underlying causes of addiction and develop effective strategies for prevention and recovery. Emphasising the importance of meaningful engagement, emotional regulation, and professional support can help mitigate the impact of boredom and reduce the risk of addiction, ultimately leading to healthier and more fulfilling lives.

CHAPTER 35

THE CONNECTION BETWEEN ADDICTION AND MOBILE DEVICES

In the modern world, mobile devices have become an integral part of daily life. From communication to entertainment, work to leisure, these devices provide unparalleled convenience. However, as usage has increased, so too has the prevalence of problematic and addictive behaviours associated with mobile phones. This chapter explores the connection between addiction and mobile devices – how it develops, why it happens, and what can be done to manage it.

The connection between mobile devices and addiction

Mobile device addiction, often referred to as 'smartphone addiction' or 'problematic smartphone use,' manifests as compulsive engagement with mobile phones despite negative consequences. This behaviour closely mirrors substance addiction, with users experiencing withdrawal symptoms, increased tolerance, and compulsive urges to check their devices.

Research suggests that mobile device addiction is driven by the brain's reward system. Social media notifications, text messages, and emails trigger the release of dopamine, the neurotransmitter associated with pleasure and reward. Over time, the brain begins to crave this stimulation, leading to compulsive checking and excessive screen time.

How it happens

Mobile device addiction does not occur by chance; it is driven by a combination of psychological, social, and technological factors. The way mobile phones and apps are designed, combined with human behavioural tendencies, creates an environment that encourages prolonged use. Understanding the underlying mechanisms can help individuals recognise their own usage patterns and take steps to regain control. Several factors contribute to mobile device addiction:

1. **Instant gratification:** Mobile phones provide immediate access to entertainment, communication, and validation (e.g., social media 'likes,' comments, and messages). The constant availability of quick rewards reinforces habitual usage. The instant nature of feedback fosters a cycle of seeking immediate pleasure, diminishing patience for delayed gratification in other aspects of life.

2. **Social validation and fear of missing out (FOMO):** Social media platforms are designed to create a sense of belonging and engagement. However, this can also lead to anxiety and compulsive checking, as individuals fear being left out of conversations, events, or trends. The pressure to stay updated and maintain an online presence can become overwhelming, leading to compulsive behaviour.

3. **Dopamine loops and algorithmic design:** Tech companies design applications to keep users engaged for as long as possible. Features like infinite scrolling, push notifications, and

autoplay videos exploit psychological vulnerabilities, encouraging users to remain glued to their screens. These algorithms analyse user behaviour and tailor content to maximise engagement, reinforcing addiction by consistently providing enticing stimuli.

4. **Work and connectivity pressure:** In a hyper-connected society, individuals feel obligated to respond to emails, messages, and calls immediately. This creates an 'always-on' culture, leading to stress and dependency on mobile devices. Many professionals find it challenging to separate work from personal life, leading to burnout and mental fatigue.

5. **Escapism and emotional regulation:** Many people turn to their phones as a coping mechanism for stress, loneliness, or boredom. This reliance can develop into compulsive behaviour, where mobile use becomes a means to avoid dealing with emotions or real-world challenges. Over time, reliance on digital distractions may hinder emotional resilience and personal growth.

The impact of mobile device addiction

Mobile device addiction can significantly affect various aspects of life, from mental and physical health to productivity and relationships. The constant engagement with screens can create a cycle of dependency that is difficult to break, leading to negative consequences that extend beyond mere overuse. Understanding these impacts is essential for recognising the seriousness of mobile addiction and taking proactive steps to address it.

Excessive mobile phone use can have profound consequences on mental and physical health, relationships, and productivity. Some of the most common negative effects include:

1. **Mental health issues:** Increased anxiety, depression, and attention problems. Overuse of mobile devices can exacerbate feelings of isolation and insecurity, particularly through excessive social media consumption.

2. **Sleep disruption:** Blue light exposure and late-night scrolling disrupt sleep patterns, leading to fatigue and cognitive impairments. The habit of checking devices before bedtime can interfere with melatonin production, making it harder to fall and stay asleep.

3. **Reduced productivity:** Constant distractions hinder focus and efficiency in both professional and academic settings. Notifications and the compulsion to check devices reduce deep work and concentration, lowering overall output.

4. **Physical health problems:** Issues like 'text neck,' eye strain, and poor posture are increasingly common. Extended screen time contributes to musculoskeletal issues, particularly in younger generations who develop poor postural habits early on.

5. **Weakened interpersonal relationships:** Face-to-face interactions suffer as individuals prioritise digital connections over real-world relationships. The lack of present-moment engagement can erode meaningful relationships, leading to social disconnection.

What to do

Recognising the negative effects of excessive mobile phone use is the first step towards breaking free from its grip. While technology is an integral part of modern life, it is possible to cultivate a healthier relationship with it. By implementing conscious habits and making intentional choices, individuals can regain control over their screen time and improve their overall wellbeing. The following strategies can help in managing and reducing mobile device addiction effectively:

1. **Recognise the problem:** The first step is acknowledging excessive mobile use and its impact. Tracking screen time through built-in phone features or third-party apps can provide valuable insights. Self-assessment quizzes can also help identify problematic patterns.

2. **Set boundaries:** Establish clear guidelines for phone use, such as avoiding phone usage during meals or social gatherings to encourage real-world connections. Implementing 'no-screen' hours before bedtime can improve sleep quality, while designating tech-free zones, such as bedrooms, promotes digital detox periods.

3. **Use technology to fight technology:** Many phones have digital wellbeing features that help users regulate screen time. These include setting app limits to control excessive usage, scheduling downtime to reduce engagement with mobile devices during specific hours, and receiving reminders when screen time exceeds set limits, reinforcing accountability. Using the 'do not disturb' mode during work or focused activities can also enhance productivity.

4. **Engage in offline activities:** Replacing screen time with alternative activities can help break the cycle of compulsive phone use. Pursuing hobbies such as reading, painting, or playing a musical instrument provides a fulfilling offline alternative. Engaging in outdoor activities, such as hiking or exercising, helps disconnect from screens while improving physical wellbeing. Strengthening real-world social connections through face-to-face interactions fosters deeper relationships and reduces dependency on virtual engagement.

5. **Practise mindfulness and self-control:** Mindfulness techniques, such as meditation and deep breathing, can help reduce the urge to check a phone unnecessarily. Practising self-discipline by resisting the impulse to check notifications immediately can gradually weaken the habit. Journaling and self-reflection can also provide clarity on emotional triggers that lead to excessive phone use.

When to seek help

For those struggling with severe mobile device addiction, professional help, such as cognitive behavioural therapy (CBT), can be beneficial. Support groups and digital detox programmes can also offer structured approaches to reducing reliance on mobile devices. Families and friends can play a crucial role in encouraging healthier habits through positive reinforcement.

1. **Impact on daily life:** If an individual's mobile phone use begins to interfere with their daily responsibilities, such as work, education, or relationships, it may indicate the need for professional help. When mobile device use starts to overshadow important activities or obligations, seeking support can help restore balance and prevent further disruption.

2. **Inability to control usage:** When attempts to reduce screen time are unsuccessful and mobile use feels compulsive or uncontrollable, it is a strong signal to seek help. If individuals find themselves repeatedly returning to their devices despite knowing it is problematic, professional intervention can offer strategies to break free from this cycle.

3. **Emotional distress:** If mobile device use is causing emotional distress, such as anxiety, irritability, or depression when not using the phone, it's important to recognise these signs

and seek help. These emotional responses can indicate an unhealthy reliance on technology, and professional support can assist in managing these feelings.

4. **Concern from loved ones:** If friends or family members express concern about the impact of mobile device use, it may be time to evaluate the situation. Loved ones may observe the extent of the problem more clearly and can provide valuable perspectives. Their concern can act as a prompt to seek professional help and begin working towards healthier habits.

Recognising these warning signs early and reaching out for help can be the first step towards regaining control over one's digital habits.

My personal experience

The constant presence of mobile devices contributed to a feeling of never being truly 'off.' The ever-pinging notifications of emails, messages and news, as well as the digital demands increased my stress levels and reduced opportunities for genuine rest. I remember being on holiday with my family one Christmas and being glued to my phone, working almost the entire time. It was horrible, for everyone. In reality, I hadn't had a genuine rest for over 17 years. I was always working when on holiday. Becoming mindful of this connection encouraged me to set boundaries and reclaim time to be present, rest, and recover.

Conclusion

Mobile device addiction is a growing concern in today's digital world. While smartphones offer many benefits, their overuse can lead to addiction-like behaviours that impact mental health, relationships, and overall wellbeing. By understanding the mechanisms behind mobile addiction and implementing strategies for control, individuals can cultivate a healthier relationship with technology, ensuring that mobile devices serve them rather than enslave them. Digital balance is key to maintaining overall wellbeing in an increasingly connected world.

By implementing strategies such as setting boundaries, engaging in offline activities, and utilising digital wellbeing tools, individuals can take control of their screen time and foster a healthier relationship with technology. Recognising the problem, seeking support, and practising mindfulness are essential steps in achieving digital balance. Ultimately, the goal is not to eliminate mobile devices; it is to ensure they serve as tools that enhance life rather than diminish its quality. Achieving a mindful approach to technology use will allow individuals to fully engage in their personal and professional lives while maintaining their mental and emotional wellbeing.

CHAPTER 36

THE CONNECTION BETWEEN ADDICTION AND SOCIAL MEDIA

In today's fast-paced world, social media platforms like Facebook, Instagram, X (formerly Twitter), and TikTok have woven themselves into the fabric of daily life. They offer endless streams of content, connection, and entertainment, often creating an illusion of productivity and social engagement. However, beneath the surface, these platforms have been found to foster behaviours alarmingly similar to addiction. This chapter explores the link between social media and addiction, delving into the psychological mechanisms that make these platforms so compelling, why people are vulnerable to them, and what steps can be taken to prevent or manage the onset of addiction to social media.

The connection between social media and addiction

The connection between addiction and social media lies in the way these platforms are designed to exploit human psychological mechanisms, creating a cycle of compulsive behaviour. Social media engages the brain's reward system by providing instant gratification through likes, comments, and notifications, triggering the release of dopamine. This constant cycle of seeking validation and social approval can lead to a dependence on social media, with users spending increasing amounts of time online despite negative consequences. The platforms also capitalise on feelings of fear of missing out (FOMO) and social comparison, further deepening the addiction. Ultimately, social media addiction mirrors other behavioural addictions, characterised by compulsive use, impaired control, and a negative impact on daily life.

The nature of social media addiction

Addiction, in its broadest sense, involves compulsive engagement in behaviours despite negative consequences. In the case of social media, addiction manifests as an inability to control the amount of time spent online, constantly checking notifications, and prioritising online interactions over real-life responsibilities or relationships. Although social media addiction is not yet classified as a formal disorder in the *DSM-5 (Diagnostic and Statistical Manual of Mental Disorders,* the standard classification of mental disorders used by mental health professionals in the United States), many of its characteristics mirror those found in other behavioural addictions such as gambling.

Social media addiction often stems from a need for validation, connection, and escapism. The platforms are designed to exploit these needs, using sophisticated algorithms to personalise content and keep users engaged. Each 'like,' comment, or share serves as a form of social approval, providing the brain with small bursts of dopamine – the chemical linked to pleasure and reward, as we have seen throughout this book. Over time, this reward system becomes reinforced, leading users to seek more frequent and intense interactions, much like substance addictions.

Chapter 36

Why social media feeds addiction

Social media is particularly potent at fostering addictive behaviours due to a combination of psychological, social, and technological factors:

1. **Instant gratification:** One of the primary reasons social media can lead to addiction is its provision of instant gratification. Users can post content and receive immediate feedback, creating a cycle of anticipation and reward that keeps them coming back. This rapid response from followers or friends taps into the brain's reward system, much like the highs experienced by those addicted to drugs or gambling.

2. **FOMO (fear of missing out):** FOMO is another significant driver of social media addiction. Users feel a compulsion to stay connected to avoid missing out on social events, trending topics, or important updates. The anxiety of being 'out of the loop' can make it difficult to disconnect from platforms, fuelling a reliance on constant engagement.

3. **Social validation:** Human beings have a natural desire to be accepted and appreciated. Social media platforms provide a constant source of social validation through likes, comments, and shares. This external validation can make users feel good about themselves, leading to an unhealthy dependence on how others perceive them online. Over time, this need for validation can grow into an addiction, as users chase that fleeting sense of approval.

4. **The illusion of connection:** Social media creates a false sense of connection, where users feel engaged with their friends and followers without truly deepening relationships. This illusion can replace real-life connections, causing feelings of isolation. Ironically, the more people rely on social media for

companionship, the more disconnected they may feel in reality, creating a cycle where they turn to platforms even more for emotional fulfilment.

5. **Endless scrolling:** Social media platforms use techniques such as infinite scrolling to keep users engaged. Without a clear stopping point, people can easily spend hours moving through content without realising it, akin to the way a gambler might continue to pull a slot machine lever hoping for a reward.

How the connection between social media and addiction forms

The connection between social media and addiction isn't purely accidental; it is, in part, by design. Social media companies employ psychologists and behavioural scientists to make their platforms as engaging as possible. They study human behaviour to create features that maximise user retention. Here are some key elements that facilitate the addictive nature of social media:

1. **Variable rewards:** Social media platforms offer unpredictable rewards, which is one of the most powerful ways to create addictive behaviour. Just as a slot machine doesn't give a payout every time, social media doesn't guarantee a reward (likes, comments) with every post or interaction. This unpredictability makes users check their phones repeatedly in the hope of receiving the next 'hit' of social validation.

2. **Personalisation and algorithms:** Modern platforms use sophisticated algorithms to curate personalised content feeds based on individual preferences and behaviours. This keeps users hooked by continually presenting content they are more likely to find engaging or enjoyable, feeding the habit.

3. **Psychological triggers:** Social media companies use psychological triggers like notifications, badges, and alerts to pull users back into the platform. These triggers often exploit anxiety or curiosity, driving users to click and engage before the feeling becomes overwhelming.

4. **The social mirror:** The constant exposure to idealised representations of other people's lives can lead to comparison, making users feel inadequate or unhappy. To counterbalance these negative feelings, they may use social media even more, seeking validation or creating curated versions of their own life that they hope will receive approval.

How to break the cycle

Recognising the signs of social media addiction is the first step to breaking free from it. Common indicators include neglecting responsibilities, anxiety when unable to access platforms, and using social media to regulate mood. Once recognised, several strategies can help manage and reduce social media use:

1. **Set time limits:** Limiting the amount of time spent on social media is crucial. Many smartphones now offer built-in time management features that allow users to set daily limits for each app. Sticking to these boundaries can help regain control over how much time is spent online.

2. **Disable notifications:** Constant notifications keep pulling users back into social media. Disabling non-essential notifications or scheduling specific times for checking apps can prevent the frequent interruptions that encourage excessive use.

3. **Engage in offline activities:** Building a rich and fulfilling offline life can reduce dependence on social media. Hobbies, exercise,

and face-to-face social interactions can help replace the need for constant online engagement.

4. **Practise mindfulness:** Being mindful of why and when you turn to social media is key. Ask yourself whether you are using it out of boredom, loneliness, or a genuine desire to connect. Becoming aware of these triggers can help break the cycle of mindless scrolling.

5. **Digital detox:** Taking regular breaks from social media - whether for a few hours, days, or even weeks - can reset your relationship with the platforms. A detox can help you gain perspective and identify whether you have been using social media in an unhealthy way.

When to seek help

While it is possible to reduce social media use on your own, there are times when additional support is necessary. If social media addiction starts to negatively impact various aspects of life, including work, relationships, or mental wellbeing, it may be an indication that professional help is needed. The following signs and circumstances suggest that it's time to seek assistance to regain control and rebuild a healthier relationship with technology.

1. **Declining work performance:** When social media use starts interfering with productivity and focus at work or school, resulting in missed deadlines, incomplete tasks, or a decrease in overall performance.

2. **Strained relationships:** If your social media habits are causing friction in personal relationships, such as frequent arguments with family, friends, or partners due to excessive time spent online or emotional neglect.

3. **Emotional distress:** Experiencing persistent feelings of anxiety, depression, loneliness, or stress directly linked to social media use. These emotions may stem from comparison, FOMO (fear of missing out), or social validation-seeking.

4. **Inability to control use:** When you find yourself unable to limit or control the amount of time spent on social media, despite attempts to cut back. This may include compulsive checking, scrolling, or feeling a constant need to stay connected.

5. **Physical health consequences:** Noticing physical symptoms, such as eye strain, poor sleep, or changes in eating habits, due to prolonged social media use. These issues can also be signs of digital burnout.

6. **Escaping real-life problems:** Using social media as a way to avoid dealing with real-life challenges or emotions. If you turn to social media to numb pain, escape responsibilities, or cope with difficult feelings, it may indicate a deeper issue.

7. **Decreased mental health:** If social media use is exacerbating mental health issues such as depression, anxiety, or low self-esteem, or if it's contributing to feelings of isolation or disconnection.

Recognising these signs and seeking professional support can help prevent further harm and allow for a more mindful, controlled relationship with social media.

Conclusion

The connection between social media and addiction is undeniable. As technology becomes more pervasive and platforms grow increasingly sophisticated, the risk of developing addictive behaviours also rises. Social media companies are unlikely to take steps to mitigate this, given that their business models rely on user engagement. Therefore, it falls to individuals to take control of their usage, recognise the signs of addiction, and adopt healthier habits.

The goal is not necessarily to abandon social media altogether; it is to engage with it mindfully, ensuring that it remains a tool for connection rather than a source of compulsion. By understanding the psychological mechanisms at play, and implementing practical strategies, it is possible to break the cycle of addiction and regain a balanced relationship with the digital world.

CHAPTER 37

THE CONNECTION BETWEEN ADDICTION AND INTERNET USE

In the digital age, the internet is a double-edged sword, providing both invaluable resources and, for some, a pathway to addiction. Excessive internet use has emerged as a pressing concern, drawing parallels with more traditional forms of addiction such as substance abuse. Understanding this phenomenon requires an exploration of the underlying mechanisms, motivations, and impacts of excessive internet usage, alongside strategies for prevention and recovery.

The connection between addiction and internet use

The digital age has revolutionised how we interact with the world; however, it has also introduced new challenges, including the rise of excessive internet use. For many, the internet serves as a tool for work, communication, and entertainment, although for some, it becomes a source of compulsive behaviour akin to addiction. This phenomenon, often referred to as internet addiction, shares striking similarities with other forms of addiction, including the activation of reward pathways in the brain and the potential for significant negative consequences in daily life. Exploring the connection between addiction and excessive internet use reveals the underlying mechanisms, psychological triggers, and societal factors that contribute to this issue, as well as practical strategies for prevention and recovery.

The nature of internet addiction

Internet addiction, sometimes referred to as problematic internet use, is characterised by an inability to control the amount of time spent online, leading to negative consequences in various aspects of life. This may manifest as compulsive browsing, gaming, social media engagement, or online gambling. Unlike physical addictions that involve substances, internet addiction is behavioural, driven by psychological rewards rather than chemical substances.

Why there is a connection

The connection between addiction and excessive internet use lies in several overlapping psychological, social, and environmental factors:

1. **Increased accessibility:** With the proliferation of smartphones and wireless internet, access to online content is virtually constant. This easy access can make it challenging for individuals to moderate their internet use.

2. **Social isolation:** Ironically, while the internet connects people, it can also lead to social isolation. Individuals may choose virtual interactions over real-life relationships, exacerbating feelings of loneliness and dependence on online activities for social fulfilment.

3. **Digital culture:** The culture of instant gratification in the digital

age fosters an environment where quick rewards are readily available. This culture can make it difficult for individuals to resist the urge to engage with the internet excessively.

4. **Mental health issues:** There is a strong link between internet addiction and mental health conditions, such as anxiety (see Chapter 21), depression (see Chapter 20), and ADHD (see Chapter 16). Individuals with these conditions may turn to the internet for comfort or distraction, leading to a cycle of dependency.

How the connection forms

Internet addiction is driven by the brain's reward system, the craving for social validation, and the need to escape reality among other factors. These factors lead to increased online engagement and dependency:

1. **The reward system:** The human brain is wired to seek pleasure and reward. Engaging in internet activities can trigger the release of neurotransmitters like dopamine, which creates feelings of pleasure and satisfaction. Over time, individuals may find themselves needing to spend more time online to achieve the same level of satisfaction, leading to compulsive behaviours.

2. **Social validation:** The internet provides a platform for social interaction and validation. Notifications, 'likes,' and comments can create a sense of belonging and approval. This social reinforcement can be addictive, as individuals crave the attention and affirmation that comes from online interactions.

3. **Escapism:** For many, the internet serves as an escape from reality. It offers a distraction from stress, anxiety, or loneliness.

The allure of immersive virtual worlds, gaming experiences, or binge-watching television series can become a coping mechanism, providing temporary relief from real-life challenges.

What to do

Managing excessive internet use requires proactive steps to regain balance and promote healthier habits. By addressing the root causes of compulsive internet use, individuals can foster a more mindful relationship with technology. Here are some effective strategies:

1. **Self-assessment:** Begin by conducting a personal inventory of internet usage. Tracking the time spent online and identifying patterns, such as the frequency or duration of online sessions, can raise awareness of excessive use. This self-reflection provides insight into areas that need adjustment, serving as the first step in reducing dependence.

2. **Set boundaries:** Establishing clear limits for internet use is vital. Set specific times when internet access is allowed, such as limiting use to work hours or setting aside 'internet-free' times, such as during meals or before bedtime. These boundaries help create a more balanced routine and reduce the temptation to engage in unnecessary or impulsive online activity.

3. **Find alternative activities:** Engage in offline activities that provide fulfilment and joy, such as pursuing hobbies, exercising, or spending time with friends and family. These activities can help shift focus away from the internet and encourage healthier, more meaningful interactions in the real world. Participating in offline experiences helps fill the void that excessive internet use might have been filling.

4. **Seek professional help:** If excessive internet use is significantly

impacting daily life, seeking professional support is a key step in addressing compulsive behaviours (see more detail in 'When to seek help' below). Cognitive behavioural therapy (CBT) and other talk therapy approaches can be highly effective in identifying the root causes of addiction and developing healthier coping strategies. This type of therapy provides valuable tools to help individuals break free from compulsive internet use.

5. **Build a support system:** Sharing your struggles with friends, family, or support groups can provide the accountability and encouragement needed to stay on track. Having a strong support network offers emotional backing, reduces isolation, and helps reinforce healthy behaviours, especially during challenging times of recovery.

When to seek help

Recognising when excessive internet use has become problematic is crucial for addressing the issue before it leads to severe consequences. Early intervention can prevent further harm and support the development of healthier habits. Here are key indicators that it may be time to seek help for internet-related issues:

1. **Neglecting responsibilities:** If internet use consistently interferes with work, school, or personal obligations, it's a clear sign of problematic behaviour. Ignoring important tasks, such as deadlines or household duties, to stay online can lead to serious long-term consequences, including loss of job or academic performance, financial issues, deteriorating personal connections or a decline in overall productivity.

2. **Compulsive behaviour:** Feeling a constant urge or compulsion to check notifications, refresh social media feeds, or engage in endless browsing is a common sign of internet addiction. The

need to stay connected or consumed by online content, often at the expense of other tasks, points to compulsive internet usage that can interfere with daily life.

3. **Loss of interest:** A noticeable decline in interest in activities or hobbies that once brought joy or meaning is another sign. When online engagement begins to overshadow real-life experiences, it may indicate a shift towards compulsive internet use, where only online interactions feel rewarding.

4. **Strained relationships:** Excessive time spent online often comes at the expense of real-life interactions, leading to strained relationships with family, friends, and colleagues. If online habits are causing distance, miscommunication, or frequent arguments with loved ones, it's essential to address this behaviour before it causes lasting damage to those relationships.

5. **Emotional distress:** Feeling anxious, guilty, or frustrated when offline may suggest emotional dependence on the internet. If a person experiences strong negative emotions or finds it difficult to cope without constant online engagement, these feelings can worsen without intervention, leading to further psychological distress and even depression or anxiety.

6. **Physical symptoms:** Extended periods of internet use can have harmful physical effects, including disrupted sleep patterns, eye strain, headaches, and/or poor posture. If these physical symptoms persist and begin to affect daily life, it's important to address the issue before it leads to chronic health problems such as sleep disorders or musculoskeletal issues.

7. **Failed attempts to cut back:** If efforts to reduce internet usage consistently fail despite a desire to do so, it indicates compulsive behaviour. This is a strong signal that professional help

may be needed to break the cycle. Overcoming internet addiction can be challenging without proper support or strategies in place.

Recognising these warning signs early can help prevent more severe consequences and support healthier, balanced relationships with technology. Seeking help at the right time can facilitate a positive change and encourage long-term wellbeing.

Conclusion

The connection between addiction and excessive internet use is multifaceted, rooted in psychological, social, and environmental factors. By understanding the mechanisms behind internet addiction and implementing proactive strategies, individuals can reclaim control over their internet use. As society continues to navigate the complexities of the digital age, fostering a balanced relationship with technology is essential for wellbeing. The journey towards recovery is challenging but attainable, paving the way for healthier habits and improved quality of life.

CHAPTER 38

THE CONNECTION BETWEEN ADDICTION AND COMPUTER GAMING

One of the most contemporary and increasingly recognised forms of behavioural addiction is the one linked to computer games. This chapter delves into the intricate connection between addiction and computer games, exploring the how, why, and what of this modern challenge, and providing strategies for mitigation and intervention.

The connection between computer gaming and addiction

The connection between addiction and computer games stems from the way these games engage the brain's reward system, offering a potent mix of dopamine-driven gratification, immersive escapism, and social interaction. Designed to captivate and retain players, games often include mechanisms like achievements, endless progression loops, and multiplayer modes, making it difficult for some individuals to disengage (see 'Why computer games have addictive potential' below). This addictive potential is heightened for those seeking solace from real-world challenges or experiencing mental health vulnerabilities. Recognising these risks and implementing strategies such as setting boundaries, fostering offline connections, and seeking professional support is essential to mitigating the impact of gaming addiction.

Understanding the nature of gaming addiction

Gaming addiction, or gaming disorder, is characterised by compulsive use of computer games, prioritising gaming over other life activities, and continuing to game despite negative consequences. The World Health Organization officially recognised gaming disorder as a behavioural addiction in 2018, underlining its seriousness. This form of addiction can manifest in various ways:

1. **Excessive playtime:** Gamers lose track of time, playing for hours or even days, often at the expense of work, study, and relationships.

2. **Preoccupation:** Gamers may have constant thoughts about gaming when not playing.

3. **Withdrawal symptoms:** Feelings of irritability, restlessness, or sadness when not able to game.

4. **Loss of control:** Inability to reduce or stop gaming despite efforts.

Why computer games have addictive potential

The connection between addiction and computer games lies in their design, the psychological rewards they offer, and the personal circumstances of the player. As mentioned in this chapter's introduction, several factors contribute:

1. **Reward systems and dopamine:** Computer games are specifically designed to stimulate the brain's reward system. Achieving goals, unlocking achievements, and progressing in levels releases dopamine, the neurotransmitter associated with

pleasure and motivation. Over time, players may become reliant on these dopamine hits, driving them to continue gaming.

2. **Escapism:** Gaming offers an immersive escape from real-world problems. For those dealing with stress, anxiety, social phobia or feelings of inadequacy, gaming provides an alternative reality where they can feel competent and in control.

3. **Social connections:** Many modern games incorporate online multiplayer modes, creating virtual communities. These foster camaraderie and a sense of belonging, which can be especially appealing to individuals feeling isolated or lonely in their offline lives.

4. **Endless engagement:** Game developers employ mechanisms like cliffhangers, daily rewards, and infinite gameplay loops to keep players engaged. These strategies exploit psychological vulnerabilities, making it difficult for players to step away.

Individuals who are most at risk

Certain individuals are more susceptible to developing gaming addiction due to personal, social, or psychological factors. These include:

1. **Youth:** Adolescents and young adults, due to their developing brains and susceptibility to peer influence.

2. **Mental health conditions:** Individuals with anxiety, depression, or attention-deficit hyperactivity disorder (ADHD).

3. **Socially isolated individuals:** People lacking robust offline social networks.

4. **High achievers in gaming:** Those who experience success and recognition within gaming environments.

What to do

Recognising and addressing gaming addiction involves a multi-pronged approach, targeting individuals, families, and the broader community. Here are some steps to take:

1. **Raising awareness:** Education about the signs of gaming addiction is crucial. Sharing information about the psychological mechanisms behind games and their impact on behaviour can help people understand the risks and take proactive steps to prevent addiction.

2. **Setting healthy boundaries:** Setting time limits on gaming sessions is an important first step. Balancing gaming with other activities such as physical exercise, socialising, and offline hobbies ensures a more balanced lifestyle. Additionally, using tools like parental controls or apps that monitor screen time can help enforce these limits.

3. **Professional support:** Seeking help from therapists who specialise in behavioural addictions can provide tailored strategies to manage gaming habits. Cognitive behavioural therapy (CBT) is particularly effective in identifying and changing problematic gaming patterns.

4. **Building resilience:** Cultivating emotional and social resilience can reduce reliance on gaming as an escape mechanism. Encouraging the development of offline connections and engaging in activities that create a fulfilling life outside the virtual world are key steps in fostering resilience.

5. **Community interventions:** Advocating for responsible game design that limits exploitative mechanics can lead to broader change. Promoting support groups for affected individuals

and their families can also provide much-needed communal encouragement and guidance.

When to seek help

It's essential to address gaming addiction as early as possible to prevent long-term harm to your health, relationships, and overall wellbeing. Recognising the warning signs of gaming addiction and seeking intervention can help you regain balance in your life. Here are key indicators that suggest you may need immediate help:

1. **Neglect of essential responsibilities:** Persistent neglect of essential responsibilities, such as work or school. This could involve missing deadlines, failing to meet obligations, or experiencing a decline in academic or professional performance due to gaming.

2. **Physical and mental health deterioration:** Significant physical or mental health deterioration linked to gaming habits. This may manifest as sleep deprivation, poor diet, lack of exercise, or increased stress, anxiety, or depression caused by excessive gaming.

3. **Strained relationships:** Damage to relationships due to prioritising gaming. Strained connections with family, friends, or colleagues often arise when gaming takes precedence over meaningful social interactions.

4. **Unsuccessful attempts to reduce gaming:** Repeated unsuccessful attempts to cut back or quit gaming. A pattern of failed efforts to reduce playtime or stop gaming altogether is a strong indicator of addiction that requires immediate attention.

Recognising these signs and seeking help can dramatically improve your quality of life and help you regain control over your gaming habits. Early intervention can prevent further harm and lead to healthier, more fulfilling relationships and daily routines.

Conclusion

The connection between addiction and computer games is a compelling intersection of technology, psychology, and social behaviour. While gaming offers numerous benefits, including entertainment, creativity, and community building, it also holds the potential for harm when indulged in excessively. By understanding the mechanisms that make gaming addictive and implementing strategies to maintain balance, individuals and society can harness the positive aspects of gaming while mitigating its risks. This journey requires collaboration, education, and a proactive approach, ensuring that gaming remains a healthy and enjoyable part of life.

PART III

RECOVERY FROM ADDICTION

The journey of a thousand miles begins with one step.

Lao Tzu, Chinese philosopher and author of the *Tao Te Ching* (6th century BCE)

CHAPTER 39

THE FOUR PILLARS OF ADDICTION RECOVERY

Addiction is an intricate, multi-layered condition that affects the body, mind, and spirit. While it manifests differently in each person, its grip can feel all-encompassing. Recovery, however, is possible for anyone who commits to the process. The foundation of addiction recovery often rests on four essential pillars: physical health, mental health, spiritual wellbeing, and social support. These pillars, when nurtured in harmony, provide the stability needed for sustained recovery and personal growth.

1. Physical health: healing the body

How: Addiction often takes a severe toll on physical health (see Chapter 11). Recovery begins with the process of healing the body, which involves proper nutrition, exercise, detoxification, and medical intervention when needed.

- **Detox and medical intervention:** The first step in physical recovery often involves detoxification. In cases of substance dependence, professional medical supervision is critical. For drugs like alcohol, opioids, or benzodiazepines, abrupt cessation can be dangerous, requiring a carefully monitored detox.

- **Nutrition and exercise:** Substance abuse often leads to malnutrition and physical weakness. A balanced, nutrient-rich diet helps restore energy levels, repair tissue damage, and strengthen the immune system. Regular physical exercise not only improves bodily function; it also boosts mood and reduces cravings by releasing endorphins, the body's natural 'feel-good' chemicals.
- **Sleep:** Re-establishing healthy sleep patterns is crucial (see Chapter 15). Many people in recovery have disrupted sleep, which exacerbates stress and anxiety. Gradually restoring good sleep hygiene supports emotional resilience and cognitive functioning.

Why it works: The body has remarkable regenerative capabilities, although recovery from addiction requires time and dedication. Physical wellbeing provides the foundation upon which emotional and psychological healing can take place. A stronger, healthier body can better resist cravings, manage stress, and support overall mental health. Moreover, addressing the physical aspects of addiction reduces many of the stressors that can trigger relapse.

Connection to other pillars: Physical health is interconnected with mental health, social interactions, and spiritual wellbeing. A physically healthy body in recovery is better able to engage with emotional challenges and connect with others, making the overall recovery journey smoother and more sustainable.

2. Mental health: rewiring the brain

How: Addiction distorts the brain's reward systems and cognitive functions. Restoring mental health requires addressing the psychological and emotional roots of addiction, as well as any underlying mental health conditions like anxiety, depression, or trauma.

- **Talk therapy and counselling:** Cognitive behavioural therapy (CBT - see Chapter 45), dialectical behaviour therapy (DBT), and motivational interviewing (MI) are all proven methods in addiction recovery. These therapies help individuals identify harmful thought patterns, learn coping mechanisms, and develop strategies to manage triggers.
- **Mindfulness and meditation:** Mindfulness practices help individuals stay grounded in the present moment and reduce impulsive behaviours. Meditation can quiet the mind, increase self-awareness, and reduce the mental noise that often leads to relapse.
- **Medication:** In some cases, medication may be necessary to support mental health, whether it's to address cravings (e.g., methadone, naltrexone) or to manage co-occurring mental health disorders (e.g., antidepressants, anti-anxiety medication).

Why it works: Addiction changes the brain's chemistry, hijacking its reward pathways and making it difficult to think clearly, manage emotions, and resist cravings. Talking therapy helps rewire the brain, fostering healthier ways of thinking and coping. Addressing mental health issues, whether caused or exacerbated by addiction, reduces the risk of relapse and promotes long-term sobriety.

Connection to other pillars: Mental health is deeply entwined with physical health, spiritual wellbeing, and social support. Improving mental clarity and emotional resilience enhances a person's ability to engage with others, rebuild relationships, and find deeper meaning in life.

3. Spiritual wellbeing: finding meaning and purpose

How: Spirituality in addiction recovery isn't necessarily about religion. It refers to a sense of connection to something greater than the self, whether it's a higher power, nature, or simply the inner self.

This pillar involves finding purpose, meaning, and inner peace, which can make recovery a transformative experience.

- **Self-reflection and journaling:** Many in recovery find that reflecting on their experiences helps them make sense of their addiction and the underlying emotional pain. Journaling is a way to process thoughts and gain insight into one's inner world.
- **Twelve-step programmes and alternatives:** For many, programmes like Alcoholics Anonymous (AA), Narcotics Anonymous (NA) or Emotions Anonymous (EA) provide spiritual guidance and a structured path to recovery. These programmes (see Chapter 41) encourage individuals to surrender to a higher power and seek personal growth through humility and service to others.
- **Personal meaning and mindfulness:** Developing a personal understanding of life's purpose can be empowering. Practices such as meditation, prayer, or spending time in nature can help individuals reconnect with their values and discover meaning beyond their addiction.

Why it works: Addiction often thrives in a state of spiritual emptiness, where individuals feel disconnected, purposeless, or lost. Spiritual wellbeing offers a renewed sense of meaning, which can fuel motivation to remain sober. It also helps address the existential pain that often lies beneath addictive behaviour.

Connection to other pillars: Spiritual wellbeing influences and is influenced by mental health, social connections, and even physical health. A person who feels spiritually aligned is more likely to approach recovery holistically, valuing their body, relationships, and mental state as interconnected parts of a whole.

4. Social support: building a strong network

How: Human connection is essential in recovery. Addiction thrives in isolation, while recovery is nourished by community and relationships. Social support comes from family, friends, support groups, and healthcare professionals, providing encouragement, accountability, and understanding.

- **Support groups:** Participating in recovery groups like AA, NA, or SMART Recovery connects individuals with others who understand their struggles. These groups provide a sense of belonging, validation, and practical tools for staying sober/on track.
- **Rebuilding relationships:** Addiction often damages personal relationships. Part of recovery involves rebuilding trust and repairing bonds with loved ones. This can take time and effort; honest communication and boundaries help create healthier, more supportive relationships.
- **Therapeutic communities and sober living:** For those in early recovery, therapeutic communities or sober-living environments offer a safe space to heal without the temptation of substances. Being surrounded by others who share the same goals promotes accountability and a sense of solidarity.

Why it works: Humans are social creatures, and support from others can make all the difference in recovery. Healthy relationships provide emotional strength, reduce feelings of isolation, and help individuals stay accountable to their goals. Having a network of people who can offer practical help, advice, or simply a listening ear, reduces the risk of relapse.

Connection to other pillars: Social support is the glue that keeps the other pillars connected. It enables individuals to better manage their mental health, find encouragement in their spiritual journey, and stay motivated to maintain physical wellbeing. Social interactions also provide the real-world feedback necessary for personal growth.

Integrating the four pillars: While each of these pillars - physical health, mental health, spiritual wellbeing, and social support - is powerful on its own, their true strength in the recovery process lies in their integration. Together, they form a holistic framework that addresses addiction from multiple angles, recognising that a sustainable recovery requires balance and harmony between the body, mind, and soul.

What to do

- **Assess and prioritise:** Everyone's recovery journey is unique. Some may need to focus more on physical health, while others might need to dive deeper into mental or spiritual healing. It's essential to assess which pillar needs the most immediate attention while maintaining balance across all four.
- **Set realistic goals:** Recovery is a marathon, not a sprint. Setting small, achievable goals helps maintain momentum. Whether it's attending a support group, improving sleep hygiene, or engaging in mindfulness practices, progress is built step by step.
- **Seek professional help:** Addiction is complex, and professional guidance is often necessary. Whether it's a therapist, doctor, or spiritual mentor, having experts on your side makes the journey smoother and more manageable.

When to implement the four pillars

Recovery can start at any point, although the sooner, the better. Every moment spent in addiction is a moment lost to its destructive grip. It's important to acknowledge that setbacks and relapses are part of the process (see Chapter 10) for many people; these do not signify failure. Recovery is a continuous journey that requires daily commitment.

Chapter 39

Conclusion

By embracing the concept of these four pillars and integrating them into daily life, recovery becomes not just an end to addiction; it is the beginning of a fuller, healthier, and more meaningful life. The journey may be long and challenging, yet with the right foundation, a life free from addiction is within reach for anyone willing to take the first step.

CHAPTER 40

ADDICTION TREATMENT: THEORY AND PRACTICE

Addiction is a complicated condition - a brain disorder manifesting in compulsive behaviours despite adverse consequences. It often involves dependence on substances such as alcohol, drugs, or nicotine, or on activities such as gambling, internet use, or eating. As we saw in earlier sections of this book, the roots of addiction lie in the interplay of genetic, environmental, and psychological factors, creating a multi-faceted challenge for treatment.

Theoretical foundations of addiction treatment

The treatment of addiction is guided by various theoretical frameworks that explain its origins and effects. Understanding these theories is essential for developing effective, tailored treatment strategies. From the biopsychosocial model that addresses biological, psychological, and social factors, to cognitive-behavioural and disease models, these foundations inform practical approaches in addiction treatment. Integrating these perspectives enables practitioners to create comprehensive, evidence-based interventions that promote lasting recovery.

Addiction treatment is grounded in several theoretical frameworks:

1. **Biopsychosocial model:** This model posits that addiction is the result of biological, psychological, and social factors. Treatment under this model addresses all three aspects, aiming for a holistic approach.

2. **Disease model:** This theory treats addiction as a chronic disease, akin to diabetes or heart disease. It emphasises the need for ongoing management and medical intervention.

3. **Cognitive behavioural theory (CBT):** This focuses on altering dysfunctional thoughts ('cognitive distortions') and behaviours. In the context of addiction, it helps individuals recognise and change the patterns that contribute to their addiction.

4. **Psychodynamic theory:** This approach explores how unresolved psychological conflicts and early experiences influence addictive behaviours. It often involves uncovering underlying issues through talking therapy.

5. **Social learning theory:** This suggests that addiction behaviours are learned through interactions with others and through observing the behaviour of role models. Treatment thus focuses on breaking these learned patterns.

Practical approaches to treatment

Implementing effective treatment for addiction requires a variety of practical approaches that cater to the individual needs of patients. These approaches range from detoxification and medication-assisted treatment to counselling and rehabilitation programmes. Each method is designed to address specific aspects of addiction, promoting not only immediate recovery but also long-term wellbeing. By utilising a combination of these strategies, treatment can be personalised to support the individual on their unique recovery journeys.

1. **Detoxification:** The initial step in many addiction treatments is detoxification, where the body is cleansed of the addictive substance(s). This process is best medically supervised to manage withdrawal symptoms safely.

2. **Medication-assisted treatment (MAT):** For some addictions, such as opioid or alcohol dependence, medications can be used to reduce cravings and withdrawal symptoms. Examples include methadone, buprenorphine, and naltrexone.

3. **Counselling and psychotherapy:** Various psychotherapeutic techniques are employed to address the psychological aspects of addiction:
   - **Cognitive behavioural therapy (CBT)** helps individuals identify and alter negative and unhelpful thought patterns ('cognitive distortions') and behaviours (see Chapters 44 and 45).
   - **Motivational interviewing (MI)** enhances an individual's motivation to change by exploring and resolving ambivalence.
   - **Family therapy** involves family members in the treatment process to address relational dynamics and support recovery.

4. **Support groups:** Peer support groups, such as Alcoholics Anonymous (AA) and Narcotics Anonymous (NA), provide a network of support and shared experience. These groups often use a 12-step programme (see Chapter 41) to help individuals achieve and maintain sobriety.

5. **Rehabilitation programmes:** These can be residential or outpatient-based and provide a structured environment where individuals can focus on their recovery. Programmes often

include a combination of talk therapy, education, and life skills training.

6. **Aftercare and relapse prevention:** Recovery does not end with treatment. Aftercare services, including continued therapy, support groups, and lifestyle coaching, are crucial for maintaining sobriety and preventing relapse (see Chapter 46).

When to seek treatment

The decision to seek treatment can be influenced by various factors:

- **Severity of addiction:** The more severe the addiction, the more urgent the need for professional intervention.
- **Impact on daily life:** When addiction begins to interfere with work, relationships, or daily functioning, it's time to seek help.
- **Previous attempts to quit:** If past attempts to quit have been unsuccessful, professional treatment may be necessary.

The role of connection in recovery

Recovery is often deeply connected to social support and relationships (see Chapter 27). Positive, supportive relationships can play a crucial role in the healing process, providing encouragement, accountability, and a sense of belonging. Conversely, negative relationships or environments can hinder progress and increase the risk of relapse.

My personal experience

I have always sensed deeply that our wellbeing is not only about the physical or mental; it is about the whole, and everything is holistically linked. In seeking a wellness reset, I found that focusing on multiple aspects of wellbeing was essential. Physical health, emotional balance, social connection, and a sense of purpose, each play a pivotal role in restoring energy and resilience. Embracing these pillars has helped me create a more holistic and sustainable foundation, which has given me greater balance and awareness.

Conclusion

Addiction treatment is not a one-size-fits-all approach. It requires a nuanced understanding of the individual's unique situation and a tailored treatment plan that addresses their specific needs. By integrating various theoretical approaches and practical strategies, treatment aims to support each individual in overcoming addiction and leading a healthier, more fulfilling life. The journey to recovery is a complex but achievable path, supported by a comprehensive, compassionate approach to care.

CHAPTER 41

THE TWELVE STEPS IN ADDICTION RECOVERY

Addiction recovery is a complex and transformative journey, and the Twelve Steps provide a time-tested framework that has supported countless individuals in overcoming their struggles with various substances and behaviours. Originally developed by Alcoholics Anonymous (AA) in the 1930s for alcohol addiction, these steps have since been adapted for a wide range of addictions, including drugs, gambling, and other compulsive behaviours. This chapter delves into the Twelve Steps, exploring their application to substance and behavioural addictions, and explaining how they work, why they are effective, and how to integrate them into your recovery process.

The Twelve Steps explained

The Twelve Steps use a specific and recognisable language that may feel unfamiliar or formal to some modern readers. Phrases such as 'We admitted...' and 'Came to believe...' appear throughout the Steps and are written in the collective voice - 'we' - to emphasise that recovery is a shared, communal journey. This language is designed to foster unity, accountability, and mutual support among those in recovery.

While some Steps refer to a 'Power greater than ourselves' or 'God as we understood Him,' the Twelve Step approach is spiritual rather than religious, allowing for personal interpretation. Whether grounded in faith, community, or inner strength, the focus is on developing a guiding force beyond the individual's immediate will. Each step encourages reflection and action, forming a structured path toward healing. Understanding the intention behind this language helps demystify the process and makes the steps more approachable for anyone seeking recovery from addiction.

1. We admitted we were powerless over our addiction – that our lives had become unmanageable

How: Acknowledge that you are unable to control your addiction to a substance or behaviour and that it has led to chaos in your life. This admission involves recognising the extent of the problem and accepting the need for change.

Why: Admitting powerlessness is the first step towards seeking help and understanding that overcoming addiction requires more than sheer willpower.

Connection: This step addresses the fundamental issue of denial, paving the way for seeking external support and recognising the severity of the addiction.

2. We came to believe that a Power greater than ourselves could restore us to sanity

How: Develop faith in a higher power or a supportive framework that can help you regain control and balance. This could be a spiritual belief, a supportive community, or a combination of both.

Why: Belief in something greater than oneself provides hope and encouragement, reducing feelings of isolation and despair in the recovery process.

Connection: This step reflects the need for support beyond personal strength, highlighting the importance of faith and community in recovery.

3. We made a decision to turn our will and our lives over to the care of God as we understood Him

How: Decide to let go of your attempts to control the addiction on your own and trust in the recovery process or a higher power for guidance and support.

Why: Surrendering control allows for a more manageable approach to recovery and reduces the burden of handling everything by yourself.

Connection: Turning over your will signifies a shift from self-reliance to seeking support, a crucial move in the recovery journey.

4. We made a searching and fearless moral inventory of ourselves

How: Conduct a thorough and honest examination of your behaviours, thoughts, and emotions related to the addiction. Identify patterns and shortcomings that contributed to the problem.

Why: This inventory provides clarity and insight into the root causes of your addiction, helping to address underlying issues and prevent recurrence.

Connection: Self-awareness is essential for growth, making this step crucial for recognising and changing harmful behaviours.

5. We admitted to God, to ourselves, and to another human being the exact nature of our wrongs

How: Share your inventory with a trusted person, such as a sponsor or therapist, and express your regrets and mistakes related to the addiction.

Why: Sharing your wrongs helps to alleviate guilt and shame, build trust, and foster accountability.

Connection: This step emphasises the role of communication and honesty in recovery, promoting a sense of relief and connection.

6. We are entirely ready to have God remove all these defects of character

How: Be open and willing to let go of character flaws and destructive behaviours that have contributed to the addiction. Prepare yourself for personal transformation.

Why: Willingness to change is essential for overcoming addiction and fosters a commitment to personal growth.

Connection: Readiness signifies a shift from recognising problems to actively seeking solutions and embracing change.

7. We humbly asked Him to remove our shortcomings

How: Make a humble request for help in overcoming your defects of character. Seek support and acknowledge your limitations.

Why: Humility allows for acceptance of help from others and reinforces the collaborative nature of recovery.

Connection: Humble requests for help reflect the ongoing need for external support and guidance.

8. We made a list of all persons we had harmed and became willing to make amends to them all

How: Identify those who have been affected by your addiction and prepare to make amends. Recognise the impact of your actions on others and plan to repair relationships.

Why: Making amends helps to rebuild trust and repair damaged relationships, fostering healing and reconciliation.

Connection: This step highlights the importance of addressing the consequences of your actions and the role of forgiveness in recovery.

9. We made direct amends to such people wherever possible, except when to do so would injure them or others

How: Approach those you have harmed with a sincere apology or restitution. Avoid making amends if it could cause further harm or distress.

Why: Direct amends help to resolve outstanding issues and demonstrate a commitment to change. Balance honesty with sensitivity.

Connection: Making direct amends is a proactive step in healing relationships and taking responsibility for past actions.

10. We continued to take personal inventory and when we were wrong promptly admitted it

How: Regularly reflect on your behaviours and promptly address any mistakes or missteps. This step involves ongoing self-assessment and accountability.

Why: Continuous self-inventory helps to prevent relapse and ensures that you remain aware of your behaviours and their impact on others.

Connection: Ongoing reflection and correction are crucial for maintaining progress and avoiding complacency.

11. We sought through prayer and meditation to improve our conscious contact with God as we understood Him, praying only for knowledge of His will for us and the power to carry that out

How: Engage in regular prayer or meditation to deepen your spiritual connection and seek guidance. Focus on understanding and following a higher power's will.

Why: Spiritual practices help to maintain focus on recovery goals and provide ongoing support and inspiration.

Connection: This step reinforces the importance of spirituality and mindfulness in sustaining recovery and personal growth.

12. Having had a spiritual awakening as the result of these Steps, we tried to carry this message to addicts and to practise these principles in all our affairs

How: Share your experiences and insights with others struggling with addiction. Incorporate the principles of the Twelve Steps into all areas of your life.

Why: Helping others and practising the principles consistently solidifies your own recovery and contributes to the broader recovery community.

Connection: This final step embodies the essence of service and integration, reflecting the transformation and growth achieved through the Twelve Steps.

Integrating the Twelve Steps into daily life

- **When to do it:** The Twelve Steps are designed to be applied continuously throughout your recovery journey. Some steps, such as making amends, may be addressed at specific times, while others, like ongoing self-inventory, should be part of your daily routine.
- **What to do:** Regularly engage with the principles of the Twelve Steps through personal reflection, spiritual practices, and support groups. Seek guidance and support from others in recovery and remain committed to the process.
- **Why it works:** The Twelve Steps provide a comprehensive framework that addresses both the psychological and spiritual aspects of addiction. By fostering self-awareness, humility, and ongoing personal growth, these steps create a solid foundation for lasting recovery.
- **What makes it happen:** The success of the Twelve Steps lies in their holistic approach to recovery, which combines self-examination, spiritual growth, and community support. The principles encourage individuals to confront their addiction honestly, seek help, and continuously work towards personal improvement.

Conclusion

The Twelve Steps offer a pathway to recovery that has been embraced by millions around the world, addressing a broad spectrum of addictions. By understanding and implementing these steps, individuals can find hope, healing, and a renewed sense of purpose. As you embark on or continue your recovery journey, remember that the Twelve Steps are not just a set of actions; they provide a transformative process that can lead to a more fulfilling and sober life.

CHAPTER 42

HELPING YOURSELF IN ADDICTION

Addiction is a complex and deeply personal struggle, one that can often feel insurmountable. However, recognising that it is possible to help yourself, even in the darkest moments, is a crucial step towards recovery. This chapter delves into how to initiate self-help in addiction, why this process is important, what makes addiction happen, and how to establish a plan for breaking free.

Understanding addiction

To understand how to help yourself, it is important to first recognise what addiction is. As the earlier sections of this book describe, addiction is a condition in which a person becomes physically or psychologically dependent on a substance or behaviour, such as drugs, alcohol, gambling, or even the internet. It alters brain chemistry, creating intense cravings and a sense of compulsion that can override rational decision-making.

As we saw in Chapter 6, addiction doesn't occur in isolation. It is influenced by genetics, environment, emotional stressors, and trauma. Many people fall into addiction as a means of coping with pain, loneliness, or overwhelming life challenges. Once the cycle begins, it becomes increasingly difficult to break because the brain's reward system becomes hijacked by the addictive substance or behaviour, creating a powerful association between it and feelings of pleasure or relief.

Why self-help is important

While external support - such as talking therapy, medical treatment, and rehabilitation programmes - is vital, self-help plays an essential role in recovery. There are several reasons for this:

1. **Personal empowerment:** Self-help encourages a sense of control and ownership over the recovery process. It shifts your mind-set from thinking of yourself as a passive victim of addiction to being an active agent of change.

2. **Day-to-day management:** Recovery is a lifelong journey, and the ability to manage cravings, triggers, and emotions on a daily basis is key to maintaining sobriety or moderation. Learning to help yourself equips you with the tools to navigate these challenges independently.

3. **Holistic healing:** Self-help can address the deeper emotional, mental, and spiritual aspects of addiction that often remain untouched in traditional treatment. By working on yourself, you can begin to heal underlying issues that contribute to addictive behaviours.

4. **Long-term sustainability:** No one can hold your hand through every moment of life. Self-help strategies offer long-term solutions that you can carry with you well beyond formal treatment, helping to prevent relapse and promote sustained recovery.

The first step: acknowledging the problem

Helping yourself begins with a simple yet often difficult step: acknowledging that there is a problem. Denial is a common defence mechanism in addiction. You might convince yourself that you have everything under control or that your behaviour isn't really that harmful. However, until you fully recognise the grip addiction has on your life, it is almost impossible to make progress.

Honesty with yourself is paramount. Take a moment to reflect on the impact addiction has had on your life. Have you faced physical health problems, damaged relationships, lost jobs, or experienced mental health struggles? Have you found yourself unable to stop using despite wanting to? These reflections can help you realise the extent of the problem.

Why addiction happens: understanding triggers and connections

Addiction rarely occurs without a reason. Often, it is a response to deeper psychological or emotional pain. Understanding why addiction happens for you personally is a key step in self-help.

1. **Trauma and emotional pain:** For many, addiction begins as a way of numbing emotional pain. This pain might stem from childhood trauma, loss, abuse, or ongoing life stressors. Substances or addictive behaviours provide temporary relief from these feelings; however, over time they reinforce a cycle of dependence.

2. **Stress and pressure:** Life's pressures - work, finances, relationships, and societal expectations - can create immense stress. For some, addiction becomes a way of coping with anxiety, fear, and overwhelm.

3. **Social and environmental factors:** Your surroundings can have a significant impact on addiction. Being in an environment where substance use is normalised, or being surrounded by others who are similarly addicted, can perpetuate the problem. Addiction thrives in environments that offer easy access to the addictive substance or behaviour.

4. **Genetics and brain chemistry:** There is also a genetic component to addiction. Some individuals are more biologically predisposed to addiction due to their brain chemistry. These individuals may experience more intense cravings and find it harder to break free from the addiction cycle.

Recognising these triggers and underlying factors can help you to better understand your own patterns of addiction. By identifying what contributes to your addictive behaviour, you can start addressing these areas directly, which will help break the connection between these triggers and the addiction.

How to help yourself in addiction

Embarking on the journey to overcome addiction can be daunting; however, empowering yourself with the right tools and knowledge is crucial for recovery. Learning to help yourself involves understanding the nature of addiction, recognising your triggers, and developing effective coping strategies. By taking proactive steps, fostering self-compassion, and reaching out for support when needed, you can regain control over your life and pave the way to a healthier, addiction-free future.

1. **Build awareness:** Self-help begins with self-awareness. Start by becoming mindful of your thoughts, emotions, and behaviours. What triggers your addiction? Is it a particular time of day, a certain social situation, or specific emotions

like boredom, sadness, or anger? Once you are aware of your triggers, you can begin to plan how to avoid or manage them. Keeping a journal can be particularly helpful. Record your thoughts and feelings when you experience cravings or engage in addictive behaviours. Over time, patterns will emerge, offering insight into what drives your addiction and how you might intervene.

2. **Set small, achievable goals:** Recovery can feel overwhelming, so it's important to set small, manageable goals rather than trying to tackle everything at once. These goals can be as simple as reducing your use gradually, replacing one addictive behaviour with a healthier one, or even attending a support group for the first time. Each small victory builds momentum and strengthens your belief that change is possible. As you achieve these smaller goals, you'll feel more confident in setting larger ones, such as complete abstinence or rebuilding damaged relationships.

3. **Develop healthy coping mechanisms:** Addiction often replaces healthier ways of coping with stress, boredom, or emotional pain. Reclaiming control over your life involves finding alternative methods to deal with these challenges. Some suggestions include:
   - **Exercise:** Physical activity can provide a natural high by releasing endorphins, which improve your mood and reduce stress.
   - **Mindfulness and meditation:** Practices like mindfulness and meditation help to calm the mind, reduce cravings, and build resilience against stress and triggers.
   - **Creative outlets:** Engaging in creative activities - such as art, writing, music, or crafts - can provide a healthy way to process emotions and fill time that might otherwise be spent on addictive behaviours.

- **Social connection:** Building positive relationships with supportive, non-judgemental people can create a sense of belonging and reduce the feelings of loneliness that often accompany addiction.

4. **Create a structured routine:** Addiction thrives in chaos. Creating structure in your day can help you regain a sense of control. Establish a routine that includes regular sleep, meals, exercise, and time for self-care. A structured routine helps to fill the gaps that addiction once occupied and provides a clear framework for your day.

5. **Seek support:** While this chapter focuses on self-help, it is crucial to understand that recovery often requires a combination of self-help and external support. Reach out to others when needed - whether that's attending a support group like Alcoholics Anonymous, confiding in a trusted friend or family member, or seeking professional therapy. There is no shame in asking for help. Sometimes, the most empowering act of self-help is recognising when you need assistance from others.

When to take action

There is no perfect time to begin helping yourself in addiction; the right time is *now*. Waiting for a major life event or a 'rock bottom' moment often leads to prolonged suffering. Taking action as soon as you recognise the problem allows you to reclaim your life before further damage occurs.

If you find yourself hesitating, ask yourself what the consequences of continued addiction might be. By envisioning a future where addiction is in control, you can motivate yourself to start the recovery journey immediately.

Chapter 42

Conclusion

Helping yourself in addiction is a courageous and necessary step towards recovery. While the path may be difficult, every small step you take in acknowledging the problem, understanding your triggers, setting goals, and building healthy coping mechanisms will bring you closer to freedom.

Self-help is not about perfection; it's about progress. It's about taking control of your life, one day at a time (see Chapter 51), and recognising that you have the power to change your story. Whether through mindful awareness, structured routines, or healthy outlets, every action you take in the fight against addiction is a victory worth celebrating.

As you move forward, remember that the process of recovery is unique for everyone. Be patient with yourself, remain committed to your journey, and take pride in every step you take towards healing and wholeness.

CHAPTER 43

DAMAGE LIMITATION IN ADDICTION

Addiction, in any form, takes a significant toll on the individual and those around them. Often, by the time the reality of addiction becomes apparent, damage has already been done – to health, relationships, finances, and even self-worth. The concept of damage limitation, or harm reduction, is essential in mitigating the negative effects of addiction, whether for the person struggling with it or for their loved ones. In this chapter, we explore what damage limitation entails, why it is necessary, and how to implement it effectively.

What damage limitation is

Damage limitation refers to strategies and actions aimed at minimising the harm caused by addictive behaviours, even if complete abstinence or recovery has not yet been achieved. It is a pragmatic approach that recognises that, while the ultimate goal may be sobriety or freedom from addiction, this is not always immediately possible. Instead, the focus is on reducing the immediate risks and long-term consequences of the addiction.

These strategies might include safer ways of engaging in the addictive behaviour (for example, needle exchanges for intravenous drug users), or methods for reducing the frequency or intensity of the addictive behaviour. Importantly, damage limitation does not condone or promote the addictive behaviour; it rather acknowledges the complexity of addiction and aims to prevent further harm until more comprehensive treatment can be pursued.

Why damage limitation is necessary

Addiction often develops over time, leaving a trail of personal, social, and financial destruction. By the time an individual is ready to confront their addiction, the damage may already be severe. Waiting for the 'perfect' moment to achieve abstinence can lead to further risks, such as:

- **Health risks:** Physical harm, such as overdose, infections, or long-term damage to organs.
- **Mental health decline:** Continued substance abuse or compulsive behaviours can exacerbate mental health conditions like depression, anxiety, or psychosis (see Chapters 16, 19, 20).
- **Relationship breakdown:** Addiction often strains or destroys relationships with family, friends, and colleagues.
- **Legal and financial consequences:** Job loss, debt, or legal problems can quickly spiral out of control as addiction takes hold.

By implementing damage limitation, it is possible to slow down or even prevent these outcomes. For instance, encouraging an individual to use drugs in safer ways may reduce their risk of overdose or infection, giving them more time to seek treatment. Similarly, providing support and education to loved ones can help maintain relationships and reduce the sense of isolation many people with addiction experience.

Chapter 43

What allows damage limitation to happen

Damage limitation strategies can only be effective when approached with a mind-set of compassion, patience, and pragmatism. Understanding that addiction is a chronic condition, and not simply a matter of willpower, is essential for implementing harm-reduction measures. A few key factors contribute to the success of damage limitation:

1. **Acceptance of the current reality:** Both the person struggling with addiction and their support network must acknowledge the severity of the situation without falling into denial. This doesn't mean giving up on recovery; rather, it means accepting that while recovery may be a goal, immediate steps can and should be taken to reduce harm.

2. **Non-judgemental support:** For damage limitation to work, the individual needs to feel supported rather than judged. Shaming or punishing someone for their addictive behaviour often leads to secrecy, further isolation, and an escalation of the behaviour. Instead, a supportive, non-judgemental environment fosters open communication and trust, which are crucial for harm reduction strategies to be implemented.

3. **Education:** Knowledge about the risks associated with addiction and the options for minimising those risks is critical. This includes understanding the physical and mental health implications of substance abuse, as well as awareness of safer practices. For example, educating someone about the risks of mixing alcohol with certain drugs, or explaining how to use clean needles, can make a significant difference in their immediate wellbeing.

4. **Professional guidance:** In many cases, damage limitation is most effective when supported by professionals – whether

doctors, counsellors, or social workers - who are experienced in harm reduction strategies. They can provide guidance on safe practices, prescribe medications that reduce the risk of overdose, or offer therapeutic support to manage cravings and triggers.

Why there is a connection between damage limitation and addiction

The connection between damage limitation and addiction lies in the very nature of addiction as a chronic, often relapsing, disorder. Full recovery from addiction is rarely a straightforward, linear process. Many people will experience setbacks or periods of relapse before achieving long-term sobriety. During these periods, the risks of further harm - whether physical, emotional, or social - are high.

Damage limitation fills the gap between addiction and recovery. It acknowledges that, while abstinence may be the ultimate goal, the road to achieving it is fraught with challenges. By minimising harm in the interim, damage limitation ensures that people have the best possible chance of surviving their addiction and eventually recovering from it.

Moreover, harm reduction helps maintain hope and momentum. For individuals who may feel overwhelmed by the idea of complete abstinence, knowing that they can take smaller steps to protect their health or wellbeing can be empowering (see Chapter 49). It keeps the door to recovery open, even during difficult times.

How to implement damage limitation

There are various methods of implementing damage limitation, depending on the specific addiction and the circumstances of the individual. Below are some practical examples:

1. **Safer substance use:** For individuals struggling with substance use, there are several harm-reduction strategies that can be applied, such as:
   - Needle exchange programmes to prevent the spread of blood-borne diseases.
   - Supervised consumption rooms, where individuals can use substances in a safer environment with access to medical help.
   - Encouraging individuals to avoid mixing drugs or drinking excessive alcohol while using substances.

2. **Medication-assisted treatment (MAT):** For addictions such as opioids, MAT involves using medications like methadone or buprenorphine to reduce cravings and withdrawal symptoms. This approach can prevent overdose and provide a more stable foundation for recovery.

3. **Mental health support:** Many people with addiction also suffer from mental health issues. Offering immediate psychological support, even before they are ready to tackle the addiction, can mitigate the emotional damage that often accompanies substance use.

4. **Financial planning:** Helping an individual set financial boundaries, such as limiting access to funds or creating a budget, can prevent the complete financial collapse that often accompanies addiction (see Chapter 24). This may also involve seeking advice on managing debt or applying for social support.

5. **Support networks:** Encouraging individuals to stay connected to a support group, whether family, friends, or a peer-based community, can reduce feelings of isolation and provide them with practical and emotional resources.

When to implement damage limitation

The short answer is: as soon as possible. Ideally, damage limitation should be introduced as soon as the addictive behaviour is recognised. This prevents the addiction from escalating unchecked and reduces the long-term consequences. However, it's never too late to implement harm reduction strategies. Even in advanced stages of addiction, when the damage may seem overwhelming, small interventions can still make a difference. For instance, teaching someone how to recognise an overdose and administer naloxone can be lifesaving.

What to do next

If you or someone you know is struggling with addiction, the first step is to reach out for help. Whether through a GP, addiction specialist, or support group, professional guidance can offer clarity on the best harm-reduction strategies. Simultaneously, educate yourself about the specific risks associated with the addiction in question and start putting basic damage limitation measures in place.

No matter how dire the situation may seem, harm reduction can provide a safety net, buying time and preserving wellbeing until recovery becomes a feasible option.

Conclusion

Damage limitation is not about accepting defeat in the face of addiction. Instead, it is about understanding that addiction recovery is often a long and difficult journey, and that protecting the individual from further harm is a vital part of the process. By recognising the importance of harm reduction, we create a space where hope, health, and recovery can flourish - even amidst the most challenging circumstances.

CHAPTER 44

UNDERSTANDING AND COMBATING ADDICTION THROUGH COGNITIVE BEHAVIOURAL THERAPY

Addiction, in its various forms, is a complex condition that affects millions of people worldwide. While it may manifest in different ways - substance abuse, gambling, internet use, food addiction - the underlying mechanisms are often surprisingly similar. In recent years, cognitive behavioural therapy (CBT) has emerged as one of the most effective treatments for addiction, providing individuals with practical tools to break free from destructive cycles. This chapter delves further into the nature of addiction, explains how and why CBT works, and provides guidance on using CBT techniques to manage and overcome addiction.

What addiction is

As outlined in earlier sections of this book, addiction is commonly understood as the compulsive pursuit of a substance or behaviour despite harmful consequences. It's driven by the brain's reward system, which becomes hijacked by certain activities that trigger the release of dopamine - a neurotransmitter associated with pleasure. Over time, the brain begins to crave these experiences more intensely, leading to a cycle of use, withdrawal, and relapse. The power of addiction lies not only in the physical dependency but also in the emotional and psychological factors that perpetuate the behaviour.

How CBT addresses addiction

CBT is based on the idea that our thoughts, emotions, and behaviours are interconnected. In the context of addiction, CBT helps individuals identify and modify the distorted thinking and maladaptive behaviours that contribute to their addiction. By challenging negative thought patterns and replacing them with healthier alternatives, CBT can significantly reduce the grip that addiction has on your life.

Why CBT is effective in treating addiction

CBT's success comes from its practical and structured approach. It tackles the mental and emotional drivers of addiction, offering strategies that empower individuals to take control of their behaviour.

1. **Breaking the cycle:** Addiction often involves a cycle of triggers, cravings, and compulsive behaviour. CBT helps break this cycle by teaching individuals to recognise their triggers and develop coping strategies to manage cravings without resorting to addictive behaviour.

2. **Cognitive restructuring:** Many people struggling with addiction hold irrational beliefs, such as 'I can't cope without this', or 'I need this to feel normal.' CBT encourages individuals to challenge these beliefs, enabling them to see their situation more realistically.

3. **Emotion regulation:** Addiction is often a coping mechanism for negative emotions such as stress, anxiety, or depression. CBT teaches skills to manage these emotions in a healthier way, without relying on substances or behaviours that reinforce the addiction.

4. **Developing practical skills:** CBT is highly practical, focusing on developing new skills such as problem-solving, assertiveness, and relaxation techniques. These skills empower individuals to handle challenges more effectively, reducing their reliance on addictive behaviours as a coping strategy.

Key CBT techniques for addiction

CBT uses specific techniques to help manage addiction, such as cognitive restructuring, behavioural activation, and mindfulness. This section introduces key methods that you can use to change your thought patterns and behaviours.

1. **Identifying and challenging thoughts:** A core part of CBT involves identifying automatic negative thoughts that contribute to addictive behaviour. For example, someone may think, 'I've had a stressful day; I deserve a drink.' In CBT, the individual would learn to challenge this thought by questioning its accuracy: 'Will alcohol really make my stress go away, or will it make me feel worse tomorrow?' This process is called cognitive restructuring and helps shift thinking patterns towards more balanced, realistic perspectives.

2. **Exposure and response prevention (ERP):** In the context of addiction, ERP is used to expose individuals to situations that trigger cravings without allowing them to engage in the addictive behaviour. For example, if someone is addicted to gambling, they might be asked to visit a casino or betting shop

but refrain from placing bets. This gradual exposure helps reduce the power of the trigger over time, allowing the person to resist their urges.

3. **Behavioural activation:** Addiction often leads to withdrawal from enjoyable or meaningful activities. CBT addresses this by encouraging individuals to re-engage in healthy activities, such as exercise, hobbies, or social events. These positive behaviours help to replace the need for addictive substances or behaviours with healthier alternatives, thereby reducing cravings.

4. **Mindfulness and relaxation techniques:** Mindfulness is increasingly being incorporated into CBT for addiction. It involves teaching individuals to become more aware of their thoughts and feelings without reacting to them impulsively. By practising mindfulness, individuals learn to tolerate discomfort, whether it be cravings or negative emotions, without immediately seeking relief through addictive behaviour.

5. **Relapse prevention planning:** One of the most important aspects of CBT for addiction is relapse prevention. This involves helping individuals develop a plan for when they face high-risk situations. A relapse prevention plan includes identifying potential triggers, developing coping strategies, and preparing for setbacks. For example, someone recovering from alcohol addiction might plan to avoid social events where drinking is a major focus and develop strategies for declining drinks when offered.

The connection between CBT and addiction

The connection between addiction recovery and CBT lies in the shared focus on the role of thought processes in driving behaviour. Addiction, at its core, is sustained by irrational beliefs and harmful cognitive distortions. For example, a person with a drug addiction may believe that they are powerless to stop, or that they need the drug to cope with daily life. CBT directly challenges these beliefs by encouraging individuals to scrutinise their thinking and develop more realistic perspectives. As individuals become more aware of how their thoughts influence their behaviour, they gain greater control over their actions, thus weakening the hold of addiction.

Steps to implementing CBT for addiction

Applying CBT to addiction involves practical steps like identifying triggers and setting goals. This section outlines how you can begin to use CBT techniques in your everyday life to manage your addiction effectively.

1. **Awareness and recognition:** The first step in applying CBT to addiction is developing an awareness of your thoughts and behaviours. Keeping a journal to track triggers, cravings, and reactions is a helpful way to start. This record provides valuable insight into the patterns that sustain the addiction.

2. **Setting clear goals:** CBT is goal-oriented, so it is crucial to set clear, achievable goals when addressing addiction. For example, rather than a vague goal like 'drink less,' a more effective goal would be, 'reduce alcohol consumption to three drinks a week.'

3. **Challenging cognitive distortions:** Once triggers and thought patterns are identified, the next step is to challenge them. This involves questioning the accuracy of harmful thoughts and replacing them with more balanced alternatives. For instance, you might replace the thought 'I can't handle stress without smoking/drinking/etc' with 'There are many ways I can cope with stress, such as deep breathing or taking a walk.'

4. **Developing new coping strategies:** As addictive behaviour is often a coping mechanism, CBT encourages the development of healthier coping strategies. This might include physical exercise, relaxation techniques, engaging in hobbies, or talking to supportive friends and family.

5. **Regular review and adjustment:** CBT is an ongoing process. As you work through the steps, it's important to regularly review your progress and adjust your approach as needed. This might involve setting new goals, refining coping strategies, or seeking additional support when faced with setbacks.

When to seek help

While CBT can be highly effective in treating addiction, it's important to recognise when professional help is necessary. If the addiction is severe, or if you're struggling to implement CBT techniques on your own, seeking help from a qualified therapist can provide additional guidance and support. Many people find that working with a therapist allows them to address underlying issues more effectively and stay on track with their recovery.

My personal experience

I found CBT fascinating. Learning how thoughts, feelings, and behaviours interact gave me a real-time understanding of what was happening under the hood of my mind. It also gave me practical tools to challenge unhealthy patterns of thinking, any time and anywhere. CBT helped me identify triggers and helped develop new responses that supported my wellbeing. I use breath work daily; it is something I have always used; now I understand why I am using it. Understanding and using CBT became a valuable part of my toolkit for resilience and sustained wellbeing.

Conclusion

Addiction is a powerful force, although it is not insurmountable. CBT offers a structured and practical approach to breaking free from the cycles of addiction by addressing the thoughts and behaviours that sustain it. Through CBT, you can learn to recognise your triggers, challenge harmful beliefs, and develop healthier coping strategies. While the road to recovery may be challenging, the tools and techniques provided by CBT, and described in Chapter 45, offer a path to lasting change, helping you to regain control of your life and achieve lasting freedom from addiction.

CHAPTER 45

COGNITIVE BEHAVIOURAL THERAPY (CBT): TECHNIQUES AND PRACTICES

As described in Chapter 44, CBT is a structured, evidence-based psychological treatment that focuses on helping individuals manage their thoughts, feelings, and behaviours. By identifying and challenging unhelpful patterns ('cognitive distortions'), CBT can significantly improve mental wellbeing and is used to treat a range of issues, from depression and anxiety to phobias and chronic pain. In this chapter, we explore how to utilise CBT techniques effectively, the practices involved, and when and why they are applied.

The foundations of CBT

As seen in Chapter 44, CBT is based on the premise that our thoughts, feelings, and behaviours are interconnected and that thoughts precede emotions and behaviours. It posits that by altering our thinking patterns, we can positively affect our emotions and actions. The approach is collaborative and time-limited, with a focus on empowering individuals to become their own therapists through self-reflection and structured activities.

Key principles of CBT

The key principles include:

- **Cognitive restructuring:** Challenging and changing unhelpful or distorted thinking.
- **Behavioural activation:** Increasing engagement in pleasurable or meaningful activities to combat negative feelings.
- **Exposure therapy:** Facing fears or avoided situations gradually to reduce anxiety.
- **Problem-solving:** Developing coping strategies for life challenges.

How to use CBT techniques

Using CBT effectively involves applying specific techniques to address and alter unhelpful thoughts and behaviours. The following sections outline practical steps to implement these strategies, highlighting how to identify, challenge, and reshape negative thinking, while building healthier behaviours.

1. Identify negative thought patterns

The first step in CBT is recognising the negative automatic thoughts that contribute to distress. These thoughts are often habitual and can be difficult to notice without practice. Common types of negative thinking include catastrophising (expecting the worst), black-and-white thinking (viewing situations as all good or all bad), and overgeneralisation (drawing broad conclusions based on a single event).

How:

- **Thought record:** This is a tool where you write down specific thoughts that arise in difficult situations. It helps to pinpoint the exact words or ideas that lead to emotional discomfort.

- **Journaling:** Keeping a diary of your thoughts can help in identifying patterns over time. Try to capture what was happening when a negative thought occurred, what the thought was, how it made you feel, and what you did in response.

Why: Understanding your thoughts is the key to changing them. By identifying negative patterns, you can start to challenge and reframe them, leading to improved mood and better decision-making.

When: Use thought records or journaling when you notice a significant change in your mood, or when you're feeling anxious, sad, or upset.

2. Challenge negative thoughts

Once you have identified your negative thoughts, the next step is to challenge them. Often, our thinking is biased or distorted, leading to unnecessary distress. By examining the evidence for and against these thoughts, you can begin to develop a more balanced perspective.

How:

- **Examine the evidence:** For each negative thought, ask yourself, 'What evidence do I have that supports this thought? What evidence do I have that contradicts it?' Often, you'll find that the thought isn't as rooted in reality as it feels.
- **Cognitive distortions:** Learn to recognise common cognitive distortions, such as mind-reading (assuming you know what others are thinking), personalisation (blaming yourself for things out of your control), or emotional reasoning (believing that your feelings reflect reality). Once you spot these distortions, you can challenge them more easily.
- **Reframe the thought:** Replace the negative thought with a more balanced, realistic one. For example, if your thought was

'I'm going to fail this project', you might reframe it as 'This project is challenging, but I've handled difficult tasks before'.

Why: Challenging and reframing negative thoughts helps break the cycle of negativity and fosters more constructive thinking patterns.

When: Engage in thought-challenging whenever you notice a negative or distressing thought that feels out of proportion to the situation.

3. Behavioural activation

A key part of CBT is addressing behavioural patterns that reinforce negative feelings. Often, when people feel anxious or depressed, they avoid activities they previously enjoyed, which perpetuates the cycle of low mood. Behavioural activation seeks to counteract this by encouraging individuals to re-engage with positive activities.

How:

- **Activity scheduling:** Plan and schedule activities that you find pleasurable or meaningful, even if you don't feel like doing them. Start small – this could be as simple as going for a walk or calling a friend.
- **Graded tasks:** Break down larger, overwhelming tasks into smaller, more manageable steps. If, for example, cleaning the entire house feels daunting, start with one room or even one corner.

Why: Engaging in activities can help lift mood and build momentum, even when motivation is low. It disrupts the cycle of avoidance and inactivity that often exacerbates mental health difficulties.

When: Implement behavioural activation when you notice that you're withdrawing from activities or isolating yourself. It's especially useful when motivation is low, or feelings of depression are present.

4. Exposure therapy

For individuals dealing with anxiety, phobias, or obsessive-compulsive behaviours, avoidance is a common coping mechanism. However, avoidance can worsen anxiety over time. Exposure therapy involves facing fears in a gradual, controlled manner to reduce anxiety responses.

How:

- **Create a fear hierarchy:** List situations that cause you anxiety, ranking them from least to most distressing. For instance, if you have social anxiety, your list might range from saying hello to a colleague to giving a public presentation.
- **Gradual exposure:** Start with the least anxiety-provoking situation on your hierarchy and repeatedly expose yourself to it until your anxiety decreases. Then, move to the next level of difficulty.

Why: Exposure therapy helps you realise that the feared situation is not as threatening as you might think and that you can tolerate the anxiety it produces. Over time, anxiety decreases, and avoidance behaviours diminish.

When: Use exposure therapy when avoidance is negatively impacting your life. Gradually confronting feared situations will reduce anxiety and improve functioning.

5. Problem solving

CBT teaches structured problem-solving techniques to help manage life challenges effectively. When faced with a problem, rather than becoming overwhelmed or reacting impulsively, you can use problem-solving strategies to address the issue calmly and constructively.

How:

- **Identify the problem:** Clearly define the problem you are facing.
- **Brainstorm solutions:** List as many potential solutions as you can, without judging them initially.
- **Evaluate options:** Consider the pros and cons of each option and choose the one that seems most feasible and effective.
- **Take action:** Implement the chosen solution and monitor its effectiveness. Adjust as needed.

Why: Effective problem-solving enhances coping and reduces feelings of helplessness, which are often linked to anxiety and depression.

When: Use problem-solving techniques whenever you are faced with a challenge or situation that feels difficult or overwhelming.

The CBT practice process

CBT is not a one-time intervention; it is an ongoing process that requires self-reflection, therapist guidance, and consistent practice. This section provides an overview of how to monitor your progress, complete homework assignments, and use CBT as a lifelong skill-building tool.

1. Self-monitoring and reflection

CBT encourages ongoing self-monitoring. This involves regularly assessing your thoughts, behaviours, and emotions to track progress and identify areas for improvement.

How: Keep using tools like thought records and activity schedules to monitor your mood and behaviour. Reflect on what strategies are working and where you may need to adjust your approach.

2. Therapist guidance and homework

CBT is typically conducted with a therapist, especially in the initial stages. However, a large component of the work happens outside of sessions. Homework is an essential part of CBT and involves practising techniques between sessions.

How: Commit to applying the techniques discussed during sessions in real life. This might involve using a thought record, engaging in behavioural activation, or completing exposure tasks.

Why: Regular practice is essential for cementing CBT techniques and translating insights into tangible change.

3. Building long-term resilience

CBT is not just a treatment for immediate problems; it is also a long-term approach for building resilience and preventing relapse. The goal is to learn skills that can be applied throughout life, allowing you to manage future challenges independently.

How: Continue to use the techniques of CBT beyond the period of formal therapy. Revisit thought records, keep scheduling activities, and confront fears when they arise.

Conclusion

CBT provides a robust framework for improving mental health by targeting unhelpful thoughts and behaviours. By understanding how your mind works and practising techniques such as cognitive restructuring, behavioural activation, and exposure therapy, you can break negative cycles and foster resilience. CBT is not a quick fix; however, with consistent effort and practice, it offers lasting tools for managing life's difficulties.

CHAPTER 46

POST-TREATMENT SUPPORT: THE PATH TO SUSTAINED RECOVERY

Addiction treatment is often viewed as a singular event – an intensive period of therapy or rehabilitation designed to rid the body and mind of dependence on a substance or behaviour. However, treatment is merely the beginning of a much longer journey. Once formal treatment ends, the need for robust post-treatment support becomes paramount in sustaining long-term recovery. Without it, the chances of relapse increase dramatically. In this chapter, we explore why post-treatment support is essential, how it works, what forms it can take, and how to build a solid foundation for continued sobriety and wellbeing.

Why post-treatment support is critical

Completing a treatment programme, whether residential or outpatient-based, marks an important milestone in recovery. However, it is not the end of the process. Addiction is not simply a matter of detoxifying the body; it is a chronic condition that deeply affects the brain's reward and decision-making systems. While treatment provides the tools for recovery, the true test lies in applying those tools in everyday life.

Post-treatment support offers a bridge between the safety of structured treatment and the unpredictable challenges of the real world. Without this bridge, individuals often find themselves overwhelmed by the stressors and triggers that previously led them to addiction. Post-treatment support offers:

- **Accountability:** Regular check-ins or meetings help maintain focus and accountability for continued sobriety.
- **Ongoing therapeutic support:** Addiction is often intertwined with emotional or psychological issues that require long-term attention.
- **Community:** Being part of a supportive network can be crucial to prevent feelings of isolation, which may trigger relapse.

What post-treatment support looks like

Post-treatment support takes many forms, tailored to fit individual needs and circumstances. The key is finding the right mix of resources that will reinforce recovery and reduce the risk of relapse.

1. **Follow-up therapy or counselling:** Regular individual or group therapy sessions allow a person to continue working through the underlying issues that contributed to their addiction. These sessions help manage triggers and develop strategies for staying sober/'clean'.

2. **Twelve-step programmes and peer support groups:** Programmes like Alcoholics Anonymous (AA), Narcotics Anonymous (NA), or SMART Recovery offer group-based support. Sharing experiences with others who are also in recovery fosters a sense of belonging, accountability, and mutual encouragement.

3. **Sober living environments:** For some, a structured sober living home offers a supportive, alcohol- and drug-free environment where they can gradually transition back into normal life while still having rules and support systems in place.

4. **Family involvement and support:** Addiction impacts not only the individual; it also impacts their family and friends. Involving loved ones in the recovery process – through family therapy or support groups like Al-Anon – helps rebuild trust and fosters a supportive home environment.

5. **Medical support and aftercare plans:** In some cases, individuals may continue to require medical support, such as medication-assisted treatment (MAT), which uses medication in combination with counselling to manage cravings or withdrawal symptoms.

The timing of post-treatment support

Post-treatment support should begin the moment formal treatment concludes. Ideally, it will have already been incorporated into an aftercare plan designed before the person leaves treatment. This plan might include scheduled therapy sessions, a calendar of support group meetings, and a list of emergency contacts for moments of crisis.

The intensity of support should be highest in the weeks and months following treatment, when the individual is most vulnerable to relapse. Over time, as they gain more confidence in their sobriety and learn how to manage stressors and triggers, the need for formal support may lessen, though it should always remain accessible.

How to build a strong post-treatment support network

Creating a personalised, robust support network is vital for sustaining long-term recovery. Here are steps to building that network:

1. **Assess needs early:** During treatment, it's important to work with therapists and caseworkers to identify what forms of post-treatment support will be most beneficial. This could include individual therapy, peer support, medical follow-up, or family therapy.

2. **Stay connected to professionals:** Regular check-ins with therapists, counsellors, or addiction specialists ensure that ongoing emotional and psychological needs are met. They can help navigate the ups and downs of recovery and adjust strategies if challenges arise.

3. **Build or join a recovery community:** Whether through twelve-step programmes or other peer support groups, being part of a community where others share similar experiences is crucial. These groups provide practical advice, emotional support, and a sense of accountability that can make all the difference during difficult times.

4. **Maintain healthy relationships:** Recovery is often a time of re-evaluating personal relationships. It's important to cultivate relationships that support sobriety and to distance oneself from toxic or enabling relationships (see Chapter 49 on Co-dependency).

5. **Focus on personal development:** Part of long-term recovery involves developing new interests and goals that replace the void left by addiction. Engaging in activities such as volunteering, exercise, or continuing education can provide a sense of purpose and fulfilment.

The connection between post-treatment support and recovery success

Research has consistently shown that individuals who engage in ongoing post-treatment support are far more likely to achieve and maintain long-term sobriety than those who attempt to manage recovery on their own. This connection stems from several factors:

1. **Ongoing skill development:** Treatment equips individuals with coping mechanisms; however, post-treatment support helps refine and apply these skills in everyday situations.

2. **Relapse prevention:** Many forms of post-treatment support focus on identifying early warning signs of relapse and teaching strategies to counteract them before they escalate.

3. **Emotional and mental health stability:** Addiction is often linked with underlying mental health conditions such as depression, anxiety, or trauma. Without post-treatment support, these issues can resurface and potentially lead to relapse. Continued therapy or counselling helps manage these conditions.

4. **Building new habits and routines:** Post-treatment support structures daily life in a way that fosters healthy, recovery-oriented habits. Whether through regular therapy sessions, group meetings, or engaging in new activities, individuals in recovery need to build routines that reinforce their sobriety.

What to do if relapse occurs

Relapse is often considered a part of the recovery journey rather than a failure (see Chapter 10). If relapse occurs, it's important to take swift, compassionate action to get back on track. Here's what to do:

1. **Seek immediate help:** Contact a therapist, support group, or sponsor as soon as possible. Having someone to talk to can prevent the relapse from deepening or becoming prolonged.
2. **Assess the cause:** Identifying the triggers or circumstances that led to relapse is crucial for avoiding future setbacks. This can be done in therapy or during a support group meeting.
3. **Adjust the recovery plan:** Sometimes, relapse signals that an individual needs more support, a change in environment, or adjustments in their aftercare plan. This may mean increasing the frequency of therapy sessions or returning to a treatment facility temporarily.

Sustaining recovery over the long term

Recovery is not a linear process. It is filled with moments of growth and moments of challenge. What makes the difference between long-term recovery and relapse is often the level of post-treatment support and the individual's willingness to continue engaging with it.

The commitment to sobriety is a lifelong journey; with the right support network, relapse can be prevented, and the path to a healthier, addiction-free life can be sustained.

My personal experience

Coming home was beautiful – and somewhat challenging. Even though I had been away to rest and reset, the real world hadn't paused. It was just like coming back from a two-week vacation, only this time something was slightly different. I knew that I wanted sustained holistic health and wellbeing. I knew I wanted positive change in all aspects of my life. Thanks to the support I had – my family, my peers, my aftercare network – I stayed steady and even enjoyed the process. It was both difficult and refreshing. The path of recovery isn't a straight line for anyone, no matter what you are recovering from. It's a daily choice, supported by people who remind you why you started on your new journey. That support made all the difference for me.

Conclusion

Post-treatment support is a vital, non-negotiable part of the recovery process. It provides the tools, community, and resources needed to transition from treatment to everyday life, allowing individuals to build a life where sobriety is not only possible; it is sustainable. The journey of recovery does not end with treatment – it begins there, and ongoing support ensures that this journey is one of healing, growth, and renewed purpose.

PART IV

SUPPORTING A LOVED ONE THROUGH ADDICTION

The good we do today becomes the happiness of tomorrow.

William James, American philosopher and psychologist, 1842–1910

CHAPTER 47

SUPPORTING ADDICTION RECOVERY

Addiction is often a solitary battle, although its impacts ripple outwards, affecting everyone close to the individual. It can send shockwaves through families, changing relationships, roles, and responsibilities. Family members might take on the roles of protector or enabler, or alternatively become distant as a form of self-preservation. These shifting dynamics can cause deep-rooted stress and resentment. Some family members may feel as though they are walking on eggshells, avoiding difficult conversations for fear of confrontation, while others may become more authoritarian or controlling in their attempts to 'fix' the problem. Understanding that addiction is a disease - not just poor decision-making - can help reset these family dynamics and foster a more supportive environment.

Family members, loved ones, and friends have a crucial role in both the recovery process and the day-to-day management of addiction. Their involvement can significantly influence the trajectory of the person's journey towards recovery.

The connection between loved ones and addiction

As we saw in Chapters 27 and 28, addiction impacts relationships in complex and deeply emotional ways. The bonds between family members or friends and the person struggling with addiction can either hinder or help their journey toward recovery. Understanding how these connections influence addiction is essential to finding the balance between love and enabling behaviour.

1. **The emotional connection:** Family members and friends often have an intimate understanding of the individual struggling with addiction. This deep emotional connection can make their support incredibly impactful. When a loved one is struggling, their relationships are often tested, and emotional bonds can both exacerbate and alleviate the addiction's effects. For example, a supportive spouse or parent can provide motivation for recovery, while strained relationships can contribute to ongoing substance abuse.

2. **The influence of familial relationships:** Addiction can alter family dynamics and the roles each person plays within the household. Family members may feel a range of emotions, from frustration and anger to guilt and sadness. Understanding these dynamics is crucial because the way family members interact with the person struggling with addiction can either support or hinder their recovery.

Why support matters

The support of family and friends can be a critical factor in the success of addiction recovery. Emotional and practical assistance not only reinforces the individual's commitment to sobriety; it also helps to reduce feelings of isolation and hopelessness. Knowing why support matters and how to offer it effectively can make a significant difference.

1. **Emotional and psychological support:** One of the most significant ways family and friends can help is by providing emotional and psychological support. This includes listening without judgement, offering encouragement, and validating the individual's experiences. Emotional support helps combat feelings of isolation and hopelessness, which are common in addiction.

2. **Practical assistance:** Support also involves practical assistance, such as helping with daily responsibilities, attending therapy sessions together, or finding and coordinating treatment options. This hands-on support can alleviate the burden of managing addiction and ensure that the individual has access to necessary resources.

How to support effectively

Offering support to someone with an addiction is a delicate balance. While love and care are vital, they must be combined with clear boundaries, open communication, and a well-informed approach. Family and friends need to understand how to support without unintentionally enabling the addiction, creating a foundation for lasting recovery.

1. **Educate yourself:** Understanding addiction is the first step towards providing effective support. Learn about the nature of addiction, its effects on the brain and behaviour, and the various treatment options available. This knowledge will help you approach the situation with empathy and informed strategies, and the core purpose of this book is to provide that knowledge.

2. **Set healthy boundaries:** Supporting a loved one does not mean enabling harmful behaviours. It's essential to set and maintain healthy boundaries to protect your own wellbeing. This includes avoiding financial support that might be used for substances, not covering up or making excuses for the individual's behaviour, and addressing any enabling behaviours.

3. **Communicate openly:** Effective communication is key. Express your concerns honestly yet gently, focusing on how the addiction affects you and the family rather than placing blame. Active listening is crucial; it ensures that the individual feels heard and understood, which can foster openness and honesty.

4. **Encourage professional help:** While emotional support is vital, professional intervention is often necessary for effective treatment. Encourage your loved one to seek help from medical professionals, therapists, and/or addiction specialists. Offer to help research treatment options, accompany them to appointments, or support them through the process of enrolment in a rehabilitation programme.

5. **Participate in therapy or support groups:** Family therapy or support groups can provide additional support and guidance. These settings offer a space to explore family dynamics, learn coping strategies, and gain support from others facing similar challenges. Participating in these groups can also help reduce feelings of isolation and provide a network of understanding individuals.

When to seek help

Recognising when it's time to seek professional help for a loved one is crucial. While family and friends can provide emotional and practical support, sometimes the situation requires the expertise of professionals. Knowing the signs, and understanding when to intervene, can prevent the addiction from spiralling out of control.

1. **Recognising the signs:** It's important to recognise when professional intervention is necessary. Signs that indicate the need for professional help include escalating substance use, deteriorating physical or mental health, legal or financial problems, and strained relationships.

2. **Early intervention:** The earlier support and intervention occur, the better the chances of a successful recovery. Waiting until the situation becomes critical can make recovery more difficult and increase the risk of serious consequences.

Conclusion

Supporting a loved one through addiction is both a challenging and rewarding journey. It requires patience, understanding, and resilience. By educating yourself, setting healthy boundaries, communicating openly, encouraging professional help, and participating in support networks, you can make a profound difference in your loved one's path to recovery. Remember, your role is not to fix the problem; it is to offer support, guidance, and unconditional love as they navigate their journey towards healing.

CHAPTER 48

THE IMPACT OF ADDICTION TREATMENT ON FAMILIES

Addiction is often referred to as a 'family disease'. While it may directly afflict an individual, its ripples extend far beyond, affecting the emotional, psychological, and even financial wellbeing of those closest to the addicted person. Family members, from parents and partners to children, often endure significant distress as they witness their loved one's struggles. The treatment process for addiction, while designed to focus on the individual, plays a pivotal role in the healing and rehabilitation of the entire family unit.

Understanding the family's role in addiction

Before delving into the impact of treatment, it's crucial to understand why the family is so deeply entwined with addiction. As we saw in Chapter 28, addiction doesn't develop in isolation; it often grows within complex relational dynamics, where behaviours and emotions become interdependent.

Families can sometimes unintentionally enable the addiction, either by trying to protect the individual or by adjusting their behaviour to compensate for the addicted person's actions. Moreover, addiction can lead to cycles of distrust, emotional distance, and communication breakdowns, which further strain relationships. Over time, family members may experience their own symptoms of emotional distress - stress, anxiety, depression, and sometimes even substance misuse themselves.

The treatment of addiction, therefore, is not solely about rehabilitating the individual; it is also about helping the family re-establish healthier patterns of behaviour and communication.

How addiction treatment can impact families

Addiction treatment is not just about the individual; it's about creating a path to healing for the entire family. This chapter covers the emotional reconciliation, improved communication, and restoration of trust that can occur when families engage in the treatment process.

1. **Emotional reconciliation and healing:** One of the most significant impacts of addiction treatment is emotional healing for the entire family. Throughout the period of active addiction, family members are likely to experience anger, frustration, guilt, and hopelessness. These emotions can deeply affect family relationships, often leading to long-standing resentments and emotional scars. Treatment provides a platform for families to address these unresolved emotions. Family therapy, a core part of many addiction recovery programmes, gives members a structured space to communicate openly, share their experiences, and begin to rebuild trust. This process can be a powerful force in fostering reconciliation, providing family members with the opportunity to better understand both the addiction and their role in the healing journey.

2. **Improved communication:** Communication is often one of the first casualties in families affected by addiction. Addicted

individuals may lie or withhold information, while family members may avoid difficult conversations out of fear of confrontation or further emotional pain. During addiction treatment, communication skills are typically a focus in therapy sessions, both for the individual and for the family. Learning how to express feelings without blame, how to listen actively, and how to set boundaries are essential tools that family members can gain during treatment. The improvement in communication not only strengthens relationships; it also reduces the risk of misunderstandings that may trigger relapse.

3. **Restoration of trust and stability:** Trust is another casualty of addiction. The secrecy and unpredictability that often accompany substance misuse erode trust between family members. This instability can leave families in a constant state of uncertainty, unsure of when or if the next crisis will occur. Addiction treatment often includes strategies to rebuild trust. With time, as the individual demonstrates sustained recovery and accountability, family members may slowly begin to trust again. Establishing consistent routines and open communication during treatment can help restore a sense of stability in the household, which is essential for long-term recovery.

4. **Relief from co-dependency:** Co-dependency (see also Chapter 49) is a common issue in families dealing with addiction. Family members may feel an overwhelming need to 'fix' or control the addicted person, often sacrificing their own wellbeing in the process. This dynamic can keep both the individual and their family stuck in unhealthy patterns. Addiction treatment often includes addressing co-dependent behaviours. Family members are encouraged to develop healthier boundaries, allowing

them to support their loved one without enabling the addiction. Learning when to step back and prioritise self-care is essential for the family's overall recovery.

5. **Financial and legal recovery:** Addiction can place an enormous financial burden on families, either through direct costs related to the addiction (e.g., purchasing substances, legal fees) or due to the loss of income from job loss. In some cases, family members may have taken on debts or faced legal issues themselves as a result of their loved one's behaviour. Treatment can mark a turning point in financial recovery. Once the individual is in recovery, they may be able to return to work, contributing once again to the family's income. In some cases, treatment programmes may offer financial counselling to help families rebuild after the chaos of addiction. While the financial recovery may take time, it's often one of the long-term benefits of the treatment process.

Why addiction treatment involves families

The family's involvement in addiction treatment is critical for a number of reasons:

1. **Addiction as a family disease:** As addiction affects every member of the family, addressing the entire family system can increase the likelihood of sustained recovery. Without involving the family, the dynamics that contributed to the addiction may remain unchanged, putting the recovering individual at higher risk of relapse.

2. **Support systems matter:** Family members are often the primary support system for an individual in recovery. Their involvement in the treatment process ensures that they are equipped with the knowledge and tools to provide the right

kind of support. This includes learning how to encourage recovery behaviours and knowing what to do if signs of relapse emerge.

3. **Breaking the cycle:** Addiction can sometimes be intergenerational, with patterns of substance misuse passing down through families. By involving families in treatment, these patterns can be identified and broken, helping to prevent future generations from falling into similar cycles of addiction.

When to involve the family in treatment

Timing is critical when involving families in addiction treatment. The right time to bring family members into the recovery process varies depending on the severity of the addiction, the treatment model being used, and the readiness of both the addicted person and their family members. Some key moments to consider include:

- **Early in treatment:** Bringing the family in early can help address urgent issues such as safety concerns, legal matters, or financial crises.
- **After detoxification:** Once the individual has gone through detox and is in the early stages of recovery, family therapy can begin to address relational issues without the influence of substances.
- **During relapse prevention planning:** Family members play a crucial role in relapse prevention. Teaching them to recognise early warning signs of relapse and how to respond appropriately can significantly reduce the risk of setbacks.

What families can do

For family members, navigating the treatment process can be overwhelming. Here are some actions they can take to support both themselves and their loved one:

1. **Seek family therapy:** Family therapy provides a safe space to address emotional wounds and build healthier relationships. It also allows family members to voice their concerns and learn about addiction in a non-judgemental setting.

2. **Attend support groups:** There are numerous support groups available for families of addicted individuals, such as Al-Anon or Families Anonymous. These groups offer emotional support and practical advice from others who have gone through similar experiences.

3. **Educate themselves:** Understanding addiction as a chronic disease can help reduce feelings of blame or guilt. Families can educate themselves about addiction, recovery, and relapse prevention to better support their loved one. This book is designed to be one way to do that.

4. **Set healthy boundaries:** Establishing clear boundaries is essential for protecting the family's emotional health and preventing co-dependent behaviours. Family members must learn when to step in and when to let their loved one take responsibility for their own actions.

Conclusion

Addiction treatment has the power to transform not only the life of the individual but the entire family. Through emotional healing, improved communication, and the restoration of trust, families can emerge from the shadows of addiction stronger and more resilient. By involving families in the recovery process, treatment offers the opportunity for collective healing, breaking the cycle of addiction, and fostering healthier, more supportive relationships.

CHAPTER 49

CO-DEPENDENCY AND ADDICTION: UNDERSTANDING THE INTERTWINED RELATIONSHIP

Addiction is a complex issue as we have seen throughout this book, and one of the least recognised yet profoundly impactful aspects of this condition is co-dependency. This psychological phenomenon often emerges in the context of addiction, perpetuating unhealthy behaviours and dynamics in relationships. In this chapter, we explore the intricacies of co-dependency, examining how it develops, why it forms such a powerful connection with addiction, and crucially, how to identify, address, and heal from co-dependent patterns.

What co-dependency is

At its core, co-dependency is an emotional, behavioural, and psychological condition that affects an individual's ability to have healthy, mutually satisfying relationships. The hallmark of co-dependency is an excessive reliance on another person for approval, identity, or a sense of purpose. In the context of addiction, this often manifests as one person becoming overly involved in the addict's life, sacrificing their own needs to take care of the addicted individual, often to the detriment of both parties.

Co-dependency can occur in any type of relationship - spouses, parents and children, friends, or even colleagues. However, it is particularly prevalent in relationships where addiction is present. The co-dependent individual becomes fixated on 'helping' or 'saving' the addict, enabling harmful behaviour while neglecting their own emotional health.

Why co-dependency happens

Co-dependency is not merely a reaction to addiction; it often stems from deeper emotional patterns and family dynamics that predate the addiction itself. Individuals who develop co-dependent behaviours often have a history of childhood trauma, neglect, or emotional abandonment. In many cases, they may have grown up in a household where addiction or mental health issues were already present. As a result, they learn to derive their self-worth from caregiving or controlling chaotic situations, believing that their value comes from 'fixing' others.

When they enter into relationships with individuals struggling with addiction, these old patterns resurface. The addict's unpredictable behaviour, emotional unavailability, and need for care align with the co-dependent's need to feel needed. This dynamic can create a powerful bond between the two, although it is built on unhealthy foundations that prevent both individuals from achieving genuine emotional freedom and recovery.

The connection between co-dependency and addiction

The relationship between co-dependency and addiction is a symbiotic one. Just as addiction is marked by compulsive behaviours and a loss of control, co-dependency is driven by a compulsive need to control or manage another person's life. The co-dependent individual may feel that their role is to 'fix' the addict, protect them from consequences, or ensure that their life does not fall apart entirely. This often leads to behaviours that enable the addiction, such as covering up for the addict, making excuses for their behaviour, or preventing them from facing the natural consequences of their actions.

This dynamic is destructive to both parties. For the addict, it removes the motivation to seek help or face the reality of their situation, as the co-dependent is constantly cushioning their fall. For the co-dependent, it leads to burnout, emotional exhaustion, and the neglect of their own mental and physical health. Furthermore, this dynamic can trap the addict in a cycle of denial, as the co-dependent person continually minimises the severity of the addiction in their attempts to 'help'.

Recognising co-dependency

Understanding whether you or someone you love is in a co-dependent relationship with an addict is the first step towards healing. Some common signs of co-dependency include:

1. **Excessive caregiving:** The co-dependent person may spend a disproportionate amount of time and energy caring for the addict, often at the expense of their own wellbeing.

2. **Difficulty setting boundaries:** Co-dependent individuals often struggle to say no, feeling guilty or anxious when they attempt to establish personal boundaries.

3. **Denial:** Both the co-dependent and the addict may deny the severity of the addiction or the unhealthy dynamics in their relationship.

4. **Control issues:** A co-dependent person may attempt to control every aspect of the addict's life, from their finances to their social relationships, believing they know what is best.

5. **Low self-esteem:** Co-dependent individuals often have a poor sense of self-worth, deriving their value from their ability to care for others rather than from within.

6. **Fear of abandonment:** Many co-dependents stay in unhealthy relationships due to a deep-seated fear of being alone or abandoned.

How to break the cycle of co-dependency

Breaking free from co-dependency is a process that requires awareness, self-reflection, and often professional help. Both the co-dependent and the addict need to address their respective roles in the relationship if genuine healing is to take place.

1. **Acknowledge the problem:** The first step is recognising that co-dependency exists. Denial is often a strong force in these relationships, so it may take time to admit the full extent of the issue. Self-honesty and openness to external feedback are crucial at this stage.

2. **Set healthy boundaries:** Establishing boundaries is essential for breaking the cycle of co-dependency. This involves learning to say no, stepping back from the addict's problems, and allowing them to face the natural consequences of their actions. While this can be challenging, it is necessary for the addict's recovery and for the co-dependent's emotional health.

3. **Seek professional help:** Therapy can be highly effective in addressing the root causes of co-dependency. Cognitive behavioural therapy (CBT), family therapy, or support groups

like Co-Dependents Anonymous (CoDA) can provide tools and strategies for changing ingrained patterns of behaviour.

4. **Focus on self-care:** Co-dependents often neglect their own physical, emotional, and mental wellbeing in favour of caring for the addict. It is important to reclaim self-worth by engaging in activities that promote self-care, such as exercise, hobbies, or spending time with supportive friends and family.

5. **Encourage independence in the addict:** It is essential to step back and allow the addicted person to take responsibility for their recovery. This does not mean abandoning them, but rather giving them the space to seek professional help, attend rehabilitation, or face the consequences of their addiction.

6. **Learn detachment with love:** One of the most difficult lessons for a co-dependent person is learning to detach emotionally without abandoning compassion. 'Detachment with love' involves recognising that you cannot control or fix another person's addiction; however, you can still offer support by encouraging them to take responsibility for their own recovery journey.

When to act

The earlier co-dependency is recognised and addressed, the better. However, it is never too late to seek help. If you recognise the signs of co-dependency within yourself or someone you care about, it is important to take action sooner rather than later. Prolonged co-dependency can lead to worsening mental health issues, including depression, anxiety, and burnout. In extreme cases, it can also escalate the addiction, as the enabler allows the addict to continue their destructive behaviours without facing consequences.

If the addict is unwilling to seek help or the co-dependent is unable to break free of the relationship's unhealthy dynamics, professional intervention may be required. An interventionist or therapist can help guide the process of confronting the addiction and addressing co-dependency in a safe and structured way.

Conclusion

Co-dependency is a deeply ingrained, often unconscious pattern that can exacerbate the destructive effects of addiction. It fosters a relationship dynamic that, while seeming to be based on care and concern, ultimately enables addiction to flourish and prevents both parties from achieving true emotional health and recovery.

Breaking free from co-dependency is not easy; however, with the right support and tools, it is possible. By recognising the signs of co-dependency, setting healthy boundaries, and focusing on self-care, both the co-dependent individual and the addict can begin to heal and rebuild healthier, more balanced relationships. Understanding and addressing co-dependency is a crucial step in overcoming addiction, for it is only by disrupting this damaging dynamic that both individuals can begin their journey towards recovery.

CHAPTER 50

THE EVOLVING RELATIONSHIP BETWEEN THE ADDICT AND THEIR FAMILY

As described in previous chapters, addiction is often referred to as a family disease, a phrase that speaks to the profound and often painful impact that substance abuse or addictive behaviours can have on loved ones. The addict's relationship with their family doesn't just change because of the addiction; it evolves in response to the complex emotional, psychological, and physical shifts that addiction brings over time. For many families, this journey can be a rollercoaster of emotions, from frustration and anger to hope and helplessness.

Understanding how this relationship changes, what drives those changes, and what family members can do is crucial in navigating the challenges of addiction. This chapter explores how the relationship between the addict and their family changes over time, why these changes occur, and what can be done to support both the addict and the family during the different stages of addiction. (Do also read Chapter 28: The connection between addiction and family life.)

The initial phase: denial and confusion

In the early stages of addiction, both the addict and their family are often caught in a web of denial. Addiction may manifest subtly at first, with behaviours that can be mistaken for stress, personal problems, or temporary lapses in judgement. Family members may not recognise the signs, or they may choose to dismiss them, believing that their loved one is simply going through a difficult period.

Why denial happens

Denial is a coping mechanism, for both the addict and their family. For the addict, admitting to having a problem would require them to confront their dependency. For the family, acknowledging the addiction means facing the fact that their loved one is struggling with something that could spiral out of control. Denial helps to preserve a sense of normality, even as the situation worsens.

The impact on relationships

During this initial phase, relationships between the addict and their family are often strained but still maintain a semblance of normality. There may be frustration, confusion, and occasional conflict; however, the fundamental bonds of love and trust are often still intact.

What to do

Early intervention is key. If family members notice unusual behaviour, it's important to approach the situation with compassion and curiosity rather than confrontation. Raising concerns early, in a non-judgemental way, can help the addict feel less threatened and more willing to talk.

Chapter 50

The escalation phase: conflict and distance

As addiction deepens, it becomes harder for the addict to maintain control over their behaviour. Substance use, or behaviour, becomes more frequent, and its impact on daily life becomes more visible. At this point, denial may give way to anger and conflict.

Why conflict arises

Family members often feel betrayed, hurt, and confused. They may lash out at the addict, attempting to force them to stop their behaviour through guilt, shame, or ultimatums. The addict, feeling attacked or misunderstood, may withdraw further into their addiction as a way of coping with the emotional intensity. This leads to increasing distance between the addict and their loved ones.

The breakdown of trust

Trust, which is foundational to any relationship, becomes a major casualty during the escalation phase. The addict may lie, hide their substance use, or manipulate those around them to support their addiction. The family, in turn, may begin to monitor the addict's behaviour obsessively, attempting to control or 'fix' the situation, often leading to further tension and resentment.

What to do

At this stage, boundaries become essential. Families must strike a balance between supporting their loved one and protecting their own wellbeing. Setting clear boundaries around acceptable behaviour - such as not enabling the addict financially, or insisting on honesty - can help prevent the cycle of co-dependency (see Chapter 49) that often develops in these situations. Seeking support from a therapist or attending family-focused addiction support groups can also be invaluable, providing families with the tools to navigate these difficult dynamics.

The rock-bottom phase: Crisis and detachment

Addiction tends to follow a downward trajectory, and for many families, there comes a point where the addict reaches 'rock bottom.' This phase is often characterised by severe consequences for the addict: loss of employment, breakdown of relationships, legal issues, and/or health crises. For the family, this is often the most painful phase, as the impact of the addiction becomes undeniable.

Why this happens

The addict's substance use has likely become their primary focus, often leading them to neglect or abandon their responsibilities and relationships. For many families, this is the moment when they realise that love, logic, and attempts to control the situation are not enough to stop the addiction. The family may feel helpless and begin to emotionally detach as a way to protect themselves from the ongoing pain.

The role of enabling and co-dependency

During this phase, family members may inadvertently enable the addiction by trying to shield the addict from the consequences of their actions. This could be through providing financial support, making excuses for their behaviour, or bailing them out of difficult situations. Enabling comes from a place of love; however, it ultimately delays the addict's moment of accountability and prevents the natural consequences of their addiction from taking effect.

What to do

Letting go is one of the hardest things a family member can do, yet it is often necessary during the rock-bottom phase. This doesn't mean abandoning the addict, but rather allowing them to face the consequences of their actions while offering unconditional love and support. Families should focus on their own self-care, seeking out therapy or support groups, such as Al-Anon, where they can find understanding and strategies for dealing with their loved one's addiction.

The recovery phase: rebuilding trust and relationships

If the addict reaches a point at which they seek help and enter recovery, the family dynamic begins to shift again. This can be a period of hope and renewal; however, it is also fraught with challenges. Recovery is not a quick fix, and it often involves setbacks, including relapses (see Chapter 10).

Why recovery is challenging for families

During recovery, both the addict and the family must learn new ways of relating to one another. The family's role, which may have been focused on managing or controlling the addiction, must now transition to a supportive yet non-controlling one. The addict, meanwhile, may feel guilt, shame, or fear about the harm they've caused and the challenges of staying sober/'clean.'

Rebuilding trust is a long process, requiring time, consistency, and patience from both sides. The family must learn to let go of past hurts and anxieties, while the addict must demonstrate their commitment to recovery through their actions.

What to do

Families will benefit from educating themselves about addiction recovery and from attending therapy or support groups tailored to their situation. Learning how to communicate effectively, how to support without enabling, and how to set healthy boundaries are all critical for rebuilding relationships.

It's also important to celebrate small victories and milestones in the addict's recovery, as this can reinforce positive behaviour and strengthen the emotional bond between family members. However, it's equally important to be realistic about the possibility of relapse and to have strategies in place to address it if it occurs.

The long-term phase: new relationships

In the long term, relationships between the addict and their family may never return to the way they were before the addiction. However, they can evolve into something stronger, healthier, and more resilient. The scars of addiction don't disappear; however, families can move forward with a deeper understanding of each other and a renewed sense of connection.

Why the relationship endures

At the core of the family dynamic is a deep bond, shaped by shared experiences and a sense of belonging. This bond, though strained, often endures even the most challenging phases of addiction. For many families, the process of overcoming addiction brings a new sense of unity and purpose, as they learn to support each other in healthier, more constructive ways.

What to do moving forward

Maintaining open, honest communication is vital to ensuring the long-term success of these relationships. Families must remain vigilant, recognising that recovery is a lifelong process and that ongoing support is essential. Continuing to attend therapy, support groups, or family meetings, can provide a foundation for this ongoing healing.

The relationship between the addict and their family will never be static; it will evolve as they continue to navigate the complexities of recovery. With time, patience, and effort, this relationship can grow stronger, built on mutual understanding, trust, and unconditional love.

Conclusion

Addiction profoundly alters the relationship between the addict and their family, but it doesn't have to destroy it. While there will be many difficult moments, families can take steps to maintain healthy boundaries, support recovery, and find healing together. Understanding the stages of this evolving relationship, and responding appropriately at each phase, can help families remain resilient in the face of addiction's challenges.

PART V

THE GUIDING PRINCIPLES OF OVERCOMING ADDICTION

Our greatest glory is not in never falling, but in rising every time we fall.

Confucius, Chinese philosopher, died 479 BCE

CHAPTER 51

JUST FOR TODAY: A GUIDING PRINCIPLE IN ADDICTION RECOVERY

Addiction recovery is often seen as a monumental task, a journey that can feel overwhelmingly vast and uncertain. For those who find themselves caught in the web of addiction, the idea of maintaining sobriety indefinitely can seem like an impossible mountain to climb. Yet, within this struggle, the practice of living 'just for today' offers a beacon of hope. Rooted in simplicity and mindfulness, this approach encourages a focus on the present moment, making recovery feel manageable and achievable - one day at a time.

Why 'just for today' works in recovery

The concept of 'just for today' is grounded in the understanding that addiction thrives on chaos, fear, and emotional instability. When consumed by addiction, individuals often feel trapped in cycles of guilt over past actions and anxiety about the future. This emotional turbulence makes long-term sobriety feel unreachable. However, by shifting the focus to what can be controlled today, individuals gain a sense of empowerment over their choices.

The power of 'just for today' lies in its simplicity. Instead of making a commitment to sobriety for a lifetime - an idea that can be daunting and even paralysing - people in recovery are encouraged to focus on staying sober for just one day. By taking things one day at a time, the path to recovery becomes more approachable. Each day becomes a fresh opportunity to make the right decisions, without the burden of thinking beyond the next 24 hours.

This daily focus builds a foundation of small successes, which, when accumulated, lead to long-term change. Every day of sobriety is a victory, reinforcing the belief that recovery is not only possible; it is sustainable.

The connection between 'just for today' and addiction

Addiction is characterised by impulsive behaviours and an inability to manage stress, emotions, or life's challenges in a healthy way. It often involves a pattern of compulsively seeking out substances or behaviours as a means of escape or relief. In this sense, addiction can create a distorted sense of time, where the individual is either constantly dwelling on past mistakes or anxiously anticipating the next opportunity to use.

The practice of living 'just for today' counters this by helping to break down time into manageable chunks. It allows individuals to regain control of their lives in a way that doesn't feel overwhelming. By narrowing the focus to today, the weight of past regrets and future worries is lifted, helping to eliminate the anxiety that so often triggers relapse.

There is also a significant connection between this practice and mindfulness, a key element in many recovery programmes. Mindfulness teaches individuals to stay present in the moment, to observe their thoughts and emotions without being controlled by them. Similarly, 'just for today' encourages a mindful approach to recovery - where the focus is on today's actions, today's choices, and today's wellbeing.

What to do: Implementing 'just for today' in daily life

To effectively implement the 'just for today' approach in recovery, it's important to build a routine around it. This is a practice that should become part of your daily life, a guiding principle that helps keep recovery on track.

1. **Start the day with intention:** Every morning, you should set your intention for the day. This could involve a brief reflection, meditation, or even saying a simple affirmation, such as 'Just for today, I will remain sober.' By starting the day with a clear purpose, you can mentally prepare yourself for the challenges ahead, with a focus solely on what can be controlled within the next 24 hours. (You can try using the 'Just for today' reading at the end of this chapter, or the Serenity Prayer on page 438.)

2. **Break the day into manageable parts:** For some, even a day can feel too long. Breaking it down into smaller parts - morning, afternoon, and evening - can make the process more digestible. During moments of stress or temptation, you can remind yourself that you only need to make it through this part of the day, reinforcing the short-term commitment to sobriety.

3. **Use reminders and affirmations:** Having physical or mental reminders of the 'just for today' philosophy can be helpful. This might involve carrying a token or card with a motivational phrase, placing post-it notes around the house, or using a mobile app to send affirmations throughout the day. These small reminders act as anchors, helping you stay focused on the present when you feel overwhelmed.

4. **Engage in mindful activities:** Mindfulness is a powerful tool in the 'just for today' approach. By engaging in activities that promote mindfulness - such as meditation, yoga, and journaling - you can strengthen your ability to stay present and calm. These activities can also serve as healthy coping mechanisms when faced with cravings or emotional stress.

5. **End the day with reflection:** In the evening, it's valuable to reflect on the day. What went well? What challenges were faced, and how were they managed? By taking a moment to appreciate the effort put into staying sober for another day, you can end the day on a positive note, reinforcing the belief that you are capable of change.

When to apply 'just for today'

The 'just for today' approach can be applied at any stage of recovery, from the very beginning to long after sobriety has been established. However, it is particularly useful during moments of vulnerability, such as high-stress situations, emotional distress, or when cravings intensify.

During these difficult times, the notion of staying sober for the rest of your life may feel overwhelming and unreachable. However, by breaking it down to the next 24 hours - or even the next hour - the goal becomes more achievable. The 'just for today' philosophy encourages all those trying to recover to take the process one step at a time, making it easier to manage the inevitable ups and downs.

This approach can also be particularly effective during early recovery, when the physical and emotional challenges of withdrawal, as well as the temptation to return to old habits, are strongest. In these crucial early days, focusing solely on today helps to prevent relapse and builds the foundation for long-term recovery.

Why 'just for today' helps: The psychological basis

The power of 'just for today' lies in the way it rewires the brain's relationship with time and decision-making. Addiction often hijacks the brain's reward system, creating a strong drive for immediate gratification, even at the expense of long-term consequences. The 'just for today' method works because it allows the brain to focus on a short-term goal – something that is both achievable and rewarding.

By committing to sobriety 'just for today', the brain is able to bypass the overwhelming thought of 'forever', while still building healthy habits. Over time, these repeated short-term successes help to rewire the brain, reducing the power of cravings and compulsive behaviours.

My personal experience

Focusing on the present day, even the present moment, has helped me manage any overwhelming feelings and reduce the pressure for perfection. It took away the stress of what was next or what I had to do and when. It gave me the ability to press pause on life and take a breath. Taking life 'just for today' became a grounding mantra that brought clarity and peace. This approach has supported me in making sustainable daily progress and continues to do so today. Living in the present moment is perhaps the most meaningful practice, as it is the only moment that truly exists in this lifetime.

Conclusion

The philosophy of 'just for today' is more than a technique - it's a mind-set that can be applied to all aspects of life, not just recovery. Whether someone is newly sober or has been in recovery for years, the ability to focus on the present moment, to make the right choices just for today, offers a sense of empowerment and freedom. It removes the burden of the past and the fear of the future, allowing individuals to take control of their recovery, one day at a time.

Ultimately, 'just for today' reminds us that change is possible, no matter how difficult the journey may seem. By embracing this principle, individuals in recovery can find strength in the present, moving closer to a life of balance, peace, and sobriety- one day at a time.

'JUST FOR TODAY' READING

The *Just For Today* reading is a widely recognised and cherished piece of literature in the global recovery community, particularly within Narcotics Anonymous (NA). Its roots lie in the early traditions of self-help and mutual support groups, echoing the simple yet profound wisdom that lasting change begins with small, daily commitments.

While its exact authorship remains anonymous, the Just For Today card was first printed by Alcoholics Anonymous (AA) in 1978; however, it was not written by AA. In fact, the card's words are slightly adapted from a regular *Boston Globe* column called 'Dr. Crane Says' that was written by journalist Frank Crane. It is generally believed that Frank Crane wrote this particular column piece in 1921. It was entitled 'Just For Today' and contained a set of 10 daily suggestions. It has today become a cornerstone in the daily practices of those seeking freedom from addiction.

Just for today I will try to live through this day only, and not tackle my whole life problem at once. I can do something for 12 hours that would appal me if I felt that I had to keep it up for a lifetime.

Just for today I will be happy. Most folks are as happy as they make up their minds to be. Just for today I will adjust myself to what is, and not try to adjust everything to my own desires. I will take my 'luck' as it comes, and fit myself to it.

Just for today I will try to strengthen my mind. I will study. I will learn something useful. I will not be a mental loafer. I will read something that requires effort, thought and concentration.

Just for today I will exercise my soul in three ways: I will do somebody a good turn, and not get found out; if anybody knows of it, it will not count. I will do at least two things I don't want to do – just for exercise. I will not show anyone that my feelings are hurt; they may be hurt, but today I will not show it.

Just for today I will be agreeable. I will look as well as I can, dress becomingly, talk low, act courteously, criticise not one bit, not find fault with anything and not try to improve or regulate anybody except myself.

Just for today I will have a schedule. I may not follow it exactly, but I will have it. I will save myself from two pests: hurry and indecision.

Just for today I will have a quiet half hour all by myself, and relax. During this half hour, sometime, I will try to get a better perspective of my life.

Just for today I will be unafraid. Especially, I will not be afraid to enjoy what is beautiful, and to believe that, as I give to the world, so the world will give to me.

CHAPTER 52

THE SERENITY PRAYER IN ADDICTION RECOVERY

The Serenity Prayer is a powerful tool in addiction recovery, revered for its simplicity and depth.

God, grant me the serenity to accept the things I cannot change,
courage to change the things I can,
and wisdom to know the difference.

Its words resonate with people facing addiction because they address both the external and internal struggles inherent in the recovery process. This chapter explores how the Serenity Prayer is applied in addiction recovery, why it holds such an important place within the journey to sobriety, and how individuals can effectively utilise it for lasting change.

Understanding the Serenity Prayer in context

At its core, the Serenity Prayer speaks to the balance between acceptance and action. For those struggling with addiction, this balance is often skewed; the need for control can become overpowering, while a sense of hopelessness may pervade situations that seem beyond control. The Serenity Prayer serves as a daily reminder that not everything in life can be influenced; however, what can be changed often lies within the individual. This acceptance is often the first step towards healing.

In the context of addiction, 'acceptance' does not mean surrendering to the addiction itself. Rather, it signifies accepting the reality of the situation - the existence of the addiction, the consequences it has brought, and the recognition that recovery requires help and commitment. Many who face addiction struggle with denial, convincing themselves they have more control over their life and behaviour than they actually do. The Serenity Prayer challenges this perception by encouraging us to accept what is out of our hands and take responsibility for what we can influence.

Why the Serenity Prayer resonates in addiction recovery

The Serenity Prayer resonates with those in recovery because it captures three essential elements needed for healing: acceptance, courage, and wisdom. Addiction often leaves individuals feeling powerless, ashamed, and confused. These feelings can lead to a deep sense of defeat or an unrelenting drive to control every aspect of life to avoid falling back into addictive patterns.

1. **Serenity (acceptance):** Serenity comes through accepting the things that cannot be changed. For those in addiction recovery, this includes accepting the past and the damage caused by addiction, recognising that they cannot go back and undo what has been done. The prayer promotes a sense of peace by encouraging those in recovery to release the grip of guilt and shame, allowing them to move forward.

2. **Courage (action):** The second line of the prayer asks for courage to change the things that can be changed. This is where the recovery process truly begins - taking action to address the

addiction. Whether through therapy, support groups, or personal growth, this courage drives the effort to create a new life. Courage also means facing the underlying issues that may have fuelled the addiction in the first place - whether these are physical or emotional pain, trauma, or mental health struggles.

3. **Wisdom (discernment):** Finally, wisdom is required to differentiate between what can be changed and what must be accepted. This is the most difficult part of recovery for many individuals. Knowing when to push for change and when to release control requires deep reflection and often guidance from others, such as sponsors, therapists, or loved ones. Over time, developing this wisdom leads to healthier coping mechanisms and better decision-making.

The connection between the Serenity Prayer and addiction recovery

Addiction is often referred to as a disease of control, as individuals seek to numb feelings, gain control over their environment, and/or escape reality. The Serenity Prayer addresses these very issues. It teaches a balanced approach to life - one that acknowledges the limits of control while empowering people to take charge of what is within their grasp. The practice of reciting this prayer can help to rewire thought patterns, offering solace and structure to those navigating the unpredictability of recovery.

The connection between the Serenity Prayer and addiction recovery also stems from its use in twelve-step programmes (see Chapter 41) like Alcoholics Anonymous (AA) and Narcotics Anonymous (NA). These programmes incorporate the prayer into meetings and personal practice because it offers a spiritual framework that is both non-denominational and universally relevant. The prayer's emphasis on surrender and action aligns closely with the steps of recovery, particularly the concept of turning one's will and life over to a higher power, whether that power is a deity, the group itself, or a sense of purpose beyond the addiction.

How to use the Serenity Prayer in recovery

In practical terms, the Serenity Prayer can be utilised in several ways to support recovery:

1. **Daily recitation:** Start each day by saying the prayer. This helps to set an intention for the day and reminds the individual in recovery of the principles of acceptance, courage, and wisdom. The morning recitation can serve as a grounding ritual, fostering mindfulness and reinforcing the values of the recovery journey.

2. **In times of crisis:** During moments of temptation, stress, or relapse, reciting the prayer can provide immediate comfort and clarity. It brings focus to what can and cannot be changed in the present moment, offering a calming effect and helping us to pause before acting on impulse.

3. **Journaling:** Reflecting on the Serenity Prayer through journaling can deepen its impact. By writing about situations in which we have had to accept certain things, muster courage for change, or seek wisdom, we can track our progress and recognise patterns in our thinking and behaviour.

4. **Guiding relationships:** Recovery often involves mending relationships damaged by addiction. The principles of the Serenity Prayer can guide these efforts, helping us to understand where we can take responsibility for healing relationships and where we must accept the boundaries and limits set by others.

When to use the Serenity Prayer

While the Serenity Prayer is often used daily, its timing can be crucial during specific stages of recovery. Early in the journey, when you are coming to terms with the extent of your addiction, the prayer can help break through the wall of denial. In these early days, acceptance is often the hardest part, and the prayer serves as a reminder that facing reality is essential.

During the middle stages of recovery, the prayer can be a tool for perseverance, especially when faced with setbacks or difficult decisions. Courage becomes vital here, as change requires consistent effort and facing the pain that may have been numbed by addiction.

In the later stages, wisdom becomes the guiding force as you navigate long-term sobriety and work towards a balanced life. Here, the prayer helps to maintain focus and manage expectations, ensuring that you remain grounded and clear-headed when faced with new challenges.

My personal experience

The Serenity Prayer offered me a way to balance acceptance, courage, and wisdom in facing challenges. Its message resonated deeply as I learned to surrender control over things I could not change while acting on what was within my power. This balance helped me cultivate deeper resilience and hope throughout my journey. It left me with a stronger sense of ease and trust in the flow of life, and a belief that everything in the universe unfolds for a reason.

Conclusion

The Serenity Prayer is more than just a set of comforting words. It is a dynamic tool in the recovery process, encouraging a balance between acceptance and change. For those facing the complexities of addiction, the prayer provides a framework for reflection, decision-making, and healing. It is adaptable to different stages of recovery and personal beliefs, making it a universal resource for those seeking serenity, courage, and wisdom.

In addiction recovery, when everything can feel overwhelming, the Serenity Prayer cuts through the noise, offering clarity and peace. It guides us towards a healthier relationship with ourselves and the world around us, where acceptance and action coexist in harmony.

THE SERENITY PRAYER

The Serenity Prayer, in its entirety, encapsulated the essence of my reset. I remember every morning, myself and the rest of the 'inmates' would all link hands and recite this powerful message together. It was a collective call for inner peace, acceptance, and courage - qualities I needed to cultivate in order to live a life of integrity and balance. As I recited this prayer, I found strength in its simplicity. It reminded me that I didn't need to control everything, and that surrendering to what is beyond my control was not a sign of weakness, it was a signal of wisdom.

God, grant me the serenity to accept the things I cannot change,

courage to change the things I can,

and wisdom to know the difference.

PART VI

THE FINAL WORD

You are the director of your life.
Be strong and live in the present moment.
Find your passion and take action today.

Oliver Rolfe

THE CONCLUSION

As we have explored throughout this book, addiction is not merely a matter of having insufficient willpower or giving way to personal weakness; rather, it arises from an intricate interplay of genetic, environmental, psychological, and social factors. It has the potential to devastate not only the individuals caught in its grasp, but also families, communities, and even entire societies.

Understanding addiction requires a nuanced approach. It involves acknowledging that, while addiction may begin with a choice - whether it be the choice to take drugs, drink alcohol, or engage in harmful behaviours - once entrenched, the compulsive nature of addiction strips away the control individuals have over their actions. The brain's reward system becomes hijacked, leading to a cycle of cravings, reinforcement, and relapse. For many, addiction becomes a chronic condition that requires ongoing management rather than a problem with a simple solution.

Throughout the various chapters of this book, we have examined addiction from multiple angles. We have discussed the biology of addiction, highlighting how substances and behaviours alter brain chemistry and neural pathways. We have also explored the role of mental health in addiction, recognising that anxiety, depression, trauma, and other psychological issues can both fuel and result from addiction. This bi-directional relationship between mental health and addiction underscores the importance of integrated treatment approaches that address the individual holistically.

Additionally, we have looked at societal factors, including the role of stigma in preventing people from seeking help. The moralistic view of addiction, often perpetuated by the media, can isolate individuals and create barriers to accessing the necessary support systems. Overcoming addiction is already an enormous challenge; the added burden of shame makes it even more difficult. A compassionate, non-judgemental approach is crucial if we are to support those struggling with addiction and guide them toward recovery.

Effective treatments for addiction exist, although they require a multi-pronged approach. Cognitive behavioural therapy (CBT), motivational interviewing, medication-assisted treatments (MAT), peer support groups, and rehabilitation programmes all have important roles. Recovery is not a linear process; setbacks are common, and relapse is often part of the journey. However, with the right combination of treatments and support, people can and do recover.

It is also essential to acknowledge the importance of prevention. While treatment is necessary for those already suffering, preventing addiction from taking root in the first place is equally vital. This means addressing the underlying risk factors, such as poverty, trauma, lack of education, and social isolation, that contribute to the development of addiction. Public health campaigns, education, and early intervention can all help to reduce the prevalence of addiction in society.

Finally, as we look to the future, there is hope. Advances in neuroscience are continually improving our understanding of addiction, leading to more effective treatments and interventions. Society's growing awareness of the need to treat addiction as a public health issue rather than a moral failing is another positive shift. By continuing to raise awareness, reduce stigma, and promote understanding, we can foster an environment where those affected by addiction are met with empathy and support rather than judgement.

Addiction is a formidable challenge; however, it is not insurmountable. Recovery is possible, and with the right support, addicted individuals can regain control of their lives. As a society, our role is to ensure that we create the conditions that allow for healing and recovery, recognising that addiction is not a personal failing but a condition that requires compassion, care, and comprehensive treatment.

Together, we can move towards a future where addiction is no longer stigmatised, and recovery is within reach for all who seek it.

THE FINALE

Looking around, there's only confusion and madness.
Here's to the present, may it bring only gladness.

Do not look to the dark, but instead to the light.
Never give up on the hardest of fights.

Life is a journey for one and for all,
And how you live it can make you stand tall.

Don't follow the crowd, instead, follow your feet.
Live your life to the sounds of your own heartbeat.

Do not follow others - let your heart be your guide.
Live to the rhythm that beats deep inside.

Life can be tough, and painful in places.
We embrace what came before us,
as this was G-d's graces.

On to the next, full of hope and belief.
Ahead full of promise and nothing but peace.

With family and loved ones right by our side,
we promise to stand strong, with nothing to hide.

With love and support giving strength to believe,
we know what must be done to follow our dreams.

We devote our lives to the ones that we love,
with guidance and strength from the powers above.

To those that have strayed, it is never too late,
to show kindness to others, and to save your own fate.

Be no preacher, no Merlin, or no magician -
we are all one people, on our own life's mission.

To onc and to all, and to all a great year.
Go into the future with hope, and with no fear.

Good luck with all that you strive to attain -
be the best you can be, through joy and through pain.

Yours sincerely, Oliver Rolfe

IF NOT ME, THEN WHO? THE BACKGROUND

While I believe I had a privileged upbringing, none more so than having a loving family and being born in London (UK), I have experienced a number of different life events that made a significant and lasting impression on me. All of these have had a very positive effect on my life and also taught me many important lessons; these include knowing that each experience we have in life comes with its own message or lesson. For me, these began when I was 5 years old...

My parents divorced, something that a very large number of families go through, especially in the Western world. Due to this, I did not spend a huge amount of time with my father growing up. I was fortunate to have a loving mother and grandparents who took the mantle in my early years. My grandfather was an important role model for me, both personally and professionally. I was extremely lucky, and I am eternally thankful to them all.

From around the age of 6 years old to date, I have had over 45 operations, most of which have required general anaesthetics, and most were at an early age (a major sinus operation at 16 left me with minor nerve damage). As someone heavily involved in sports, I had a few injuries that needed other operations: a broken arm, snapped wrist, damaged knee cartilage, and ankle and foot damage.

I also suffered with asthma, which made it more difficult to play the sports I loved to be involved in daily. I lost quite a bit of time at school as a result of the operations and recovery time. That said, I was always in either the first or second team for every sport I played (about five), and usually as captain. It was something that happened, and something I always enjoyed.

At the age of 13, I was what you would call… 'fat', a word I hate to use. I was around 50 pounds heavier than I am now. I was called names, though never harshly. Being sporty as I've described, helped more than anything else. To be fair, I am not sure I really cared about my weight until I was about 16, when the other sex became visible to me. Being big at that time has always stayed with me, and I certainly eat a lot differently now to how I used to. My family love to remind me of the number of pizzas and hot dogs I ate. What can I say? I like my food. Still do!

Around that time, between the ages of 18 and 20, I suffered from glandular fever and chronic fatigue syndrome. This was a short time after I had left school and was working for an accountancy firm (BDO Stoy Hayward). I remember having constantly low energy; however, I never over-thought it and managed to use my focus on the work to find me the energy I needed. I know that sounds easier said than done; it is! Both glandular fever and chronic fatigue syndrome can be debilitating for many people.

During my upbringing, after the divorce of my parents, my siblings had their own personal difficulties. I remember different parts of these times, and I am delighted to see the strength, drive, and passion of them both, as well as the success it has brought to them.

Around the same time that my siblings were going through their own difficulties, I had a difficult relationship with a girl I loved dearly, who was from another country. After nearly three years of an intense relationship, we separated, and she returned home. It was then that she told me she had fallen pregnant, with my child (something I never truly believed). Three years later the truth came out and the child was not mine. This was a situation I had to deal with alone at the time. My family was focusing on helping my siblings and I did not want them to have any additional stress. Unfortunately, this had an effect on other relationships around me for some years, until I discovered the truth. As I am sure you can appreciate. This is something I do not blame anyone for. I have come to realise that we all have our reasons at the time for making certain decisions. We are still learning; we will always be learning.

Moving on...

At 32 I slipped a disc in my back and had to wear a metal brace for six months. This made me look like a poor man's Iron Man, rather than anything else. At that time, I was deeply concerned that I would never be able to carry my children or play with them in the park again. That was a tough moment. The only way to get through situations like that is to take one day at a time. We can never look too far into the future and be obsessed with what might be. We can only ever affect this present moment. This present moment is the ONLY one that exists.

One small step at a time. One foot in front of the other.

More recently, it has been found that I have a total of seven damaged discs throughout my spine and I have been diagnosed with something called non-radiographic ankylosing spondylitis (an inflammatory disease of the spine). This is most certainly another experience to go through, and something to learn from and assist others with. I am fortunate to be under very good medical care and will continue to progress positively.

Two life-changing experiences

While I have detailed some of the struggles that we will all encounter in our lives, and specifically those that I have already ventured through myself, I have failed to mention two life events that could have immediately changed, or shall I say halted, my life forever.

When I was around 3 years old, my family (Mum, Dad, brother, sister and family friends) and I were out for the day at Regent's Park in London. From what I remember and have in mind, it was a beautiful day and we were so happy being together. We decided that we would all go on one of the rowing boats in the lake, something I had never done before. As the attendant held the boat for us, my dad stepped onto it first, followed by my sister and then me. We were all ready to go, while enjoying the sights of the sunny park, waiting for my mother to join us in the boat. As she put her first foot in the boat, for some reason the attendant let it move away from the siding; she was caught somewhere between the side edge and the boat, almost doing the splits. All of a sudden, the boat flipped over and we capsized. From what I was told, my dad managed to get to the side and pull himself out of the water, my sister was able to swim away from the boat, and I... I was stuck underneath the capsized boat. Even now all I can remember is darkness. No sounds, no lights, just pure, black, darkness. I was going to drown! I still have no idea for how long I was under the boat; all I do know is that my 7-year-old sister went under the water, and under the boat to find me. Somehow, she managed to grab me and pull me out from under the boat and again from under the water. At that moment, I remember my father grabbing me by my lake-soaked clothes and pulling me out of the water. Had my sister not had the immediate reaction she did, this story could have turned from a dramatic anecdote to one of tragedy. I am not only fortunate to have a sister who was willing to put herself in harm's way; I am fortunate that there were no forwarding issues, barring the fact that I am not a big fan of going on rowing boats, or any boats as a matter of fact. It also taught me the importance of being a strong swimmer.

We never quite know when our time will be up on the earth plane; however, we have to ensure that we make the most out of every opportunity we have, appreciate all that is around us, and take nothing for granted.

The second life-changing experience happened when I was 7 or 8 years old. I had to go through a number of operations, as I've already described. At one time, I had two general anaesthetic operations within three months for the same issue.

Whenever you have an operation, you are either wheeled down in a bed or wheelchair to the anaesthetist's room, which is connected to the operating theatre, or asked to walk. I always hated walking down; it felt worse. I would always try and calm my nerves, whether walking or being wheeled down in a bed; however, I would always arrive with fear. I remember lying in the anaesthetist's room on the operating table; it was always so, so cold in those rooms, it felt like a fridge and usually made my teeth chatter. My mother was next to me, for comfort, as I lay on the table ready to be put to sleep. I never enjoyed that much as a child, as I am sure you can imagine. The anaesthesia of choice as a child was gas, for which they used a gas mask, something I also hated. I still remember this so clearly... I really detested the smell and taste of the gas, so I took in the biggest breath I could, and I held it. The issue with holding my breath was that I had taken in a big gulp of the anaesthetic gas, and it was putting me to sleep without my breathing. I remember slipping out of consciousness; that was where the problem started. My mother recalls standing next me, with me apparently asleep, and suddenly I started to turn blue. The reality was that I had stopped breathing completely and was now unconscious. She pointed this out to the surgeons who were preparing for my operation. At this point my mother was quickly ushered out of the room before they began to resuscitate me and get me breathing again. Had it not been for her standing there, who knows what would have happened. I could have suffered a myriad of ills, or worse, not been here to tell the tale.

My response to what life brings

It is safe to say that I have packed a lifetime of experiences into just a few decades. Indeed, you could say that I have lived a life filled with diverse experiences - personal, physical, mental, emotional, and spiritual - that have not only shaped who I am but also how I view life and the world. These experiences have driven me to explore how much more we can do to support and uplift others.

One key lesson I have learned is the importance of gratitude. It is all too easy to focus on what we lack, often overlooking all the good that surrounds us - be it good health, a loving family, fulfilling work, or even the simple pleasures like a beautiful sunset, the changing leaves of autumn, a warm meal, or a safe place to sleep. By appreciating what we have, we can approach life more positively and focus on changing what is within our control, while accepting what lies beyond it.

In writing this book and my earlier books, I have drawn on the works of some of the world's most respected scientists, doctors, and other leading minds. I have had the support of a psychologist with 30 years of professional experience, an international numerologist, a healer/medium, and the CEO of an addiction and wellness rehabilitation centre. However, despite the success of my second book on health and wellbeing, I failed to follow my own advice. I reached a point where I needed to undergo a wellness reset programme at Steps Together's Rainford Hall for over two weeks, as

I've described at the start of the book. My downfall was poor health, pushing myself to the extreme in my work, and juggling the ups and downs of family life. This included packing 22 meetings into just four days during a trip to New York City, waking up at 4:30 AM due to jet lag, and then working through a relentless schedule of meetings, followed by late-afternoon drinks and dinners. This lifestyle was typical throughout my more than 20-year career, particularly since starting my own company over 15 years ago. On top of this, I juggled the complexities of family life: raising two children with ADHD, supporting a grieving wife after the loss of her father, managing a strained relationship with my own father, and constantly being there for others. In all this, I completely neglected myself. And it almost cost me my life.

My physical and mental health deteriorated. I lost touch with my family, friends, and, most tragically, with myself. I no longer knew who I was or what I enjoyed. The irony of writing a successful book on health and wellbeing, while neglecting my own health and mental wellbeing, was not lost on me.

Through this journey, I have come to deeply understand the importance of recognising when to ask for help, being aware of what is happening within you, identifying the signs of distress, speaking your truth, and confronting difficult situations or relationships. It is vital not to bury your head in the sand or to use alcohol, drugs, medication, overworking, shopping, exercising, or any other addictions to numb your feelings or make you feel better.

I ignored these signs for far too long, and it nearly cost me everything – my business, my family, my friends, and ultimately, my life.

Many of us strive to help others navigate the storms of life. However, I urge you to pay attention to your own warning signs, no matter how challenging they may be – because if you don't, you won't be there to help anyone else. We never know when our time is up, yet we can make the most of every moment. Life is fragile, and in an instant, everything can change. That's why it's crucial to seize the day and pursue your dreams with purpose.

Take nothing for granted and appreciate the small things in life.

Make your dreams and aspirations your reality.

Take Action Today!

BIBLIOGRAPHY

PART I: UNDERSTANDING ADDICTION

Chapter 1: Why did addiction happen to me?

Books

West R. *Theory of Addiction (2nd ed).* Wiley-Blackwell; 2013.

Journal articles

Koob GF, Volkow ND. Neurobiology of Addiction: A Hedonic Calvinist View. *Philosophical Transactions of the Royal Society B: Biological Sciences* 2016; 371(1706): 20150107.

Volkow ND, Koob GF, McLellan AT. Neurobiologic Advances from the Brain Disease Model of Addiction. *New England Journal of Medicine* 2016; 374(4), 363-371. doi:10.1056/NEJMra1511480

Online resources

National Institute on Drug Abuse (NIDA). Understanding Drug Use and Addiction. National Institute on Drug Abuse. NIDA; 2020. www.drugabuse.gov/publications/drugfacts/understanding-drug-use-addiction (Accessed 10 September 2024)

Chapter 2: Breaking the stigma of addiction

Journal articles

Corrigan PW, Watson AC. The stigma of psychiatric disorders and the public's role in the mental health system. *Journal of Social Issues* 2002; 58(2): 551-567. doi:10.1111/1540-4560.00270

Room R. Stigma, social inequality and alcohol and drug use. *Drug and Alcohol Review* 2005; 24(2): 143-155. doi:10.1080/09595230500122859

Online resources

National Institute on Drug Abuse (NIDA). Stigma and Discrimination. NIDA; 2021. https://nida.nih.gov/research-topics/stigma-discrimination (Accessed 28 July 2025)

Chapter 3: The how, what, when, and why of addiction

Books

Koob GF, Arends MA, Le Moal M. *Drugs, Addiction, and the Brain.* Academic Press; 2014.

Marlatt GA, Donovan DM. *Relapse Prevention: Maintenance Strategies in the Treatment of Addictive Behaviours*. The Guilford Press; 2005.

Maté G. *In the Realm of Hungry Ghosts: Close Encounters with Addiction.* Knopf Canada; 2008.

Journal articles

Robinson TE, Berridge KC. Addiction. *Annual Review of Psychology* 2003; 54: 25-53.

Sinha R. Chronic Stress, Drug Use, and Vulnerability to Addiction. *Annals of the New York Academy of Sciences* 2008; 1141(1), 105-130.

Volkow ND, Koob GF, McLellan AT. Neurobiologic Advances from the Brain Disease Model of Addiction. New England Journal of Medicine, 2016; 374(4): 363-371.

Volkow ND, Li TK. The Neuroscience of Addiction. *Nature Neuroscience* 2005; 8(11): 1429-1430.

Reports

National Institute on Drug Abuse (NIDA) Drugs, Brains, and Behaviour: The Science of Addiction. NIDA; 2020. www.drugabuse.gov (Accessed 3 May 2025)

Substance Abuse and Mental Health Services Administration (SAMHSA). The Treatment of Addiction: What Families Need to Know. SAMHSA; 2021. www.samhsa.gov/find-support/learn-about-treatment (Accessed 3 May 2025)

World Health Organization (WHO). Neuroscience of Psychoactive Substance Use and Dependence. Geneva: WHO; 2004. https://www.who.int/publications/i/item/neuroscience-of-psychoactive-substance-use-and-dependence (Accessed 28 July 2025)

Chapter 4: The five characteristics of addiction

Books

McMurran, M. *Addiction: Psychology and Treatment.* Wiley-Blackwell; 2012.

West R, Brown J. *Theory of Addiction (2nd ed).* Wiley-Blackwell; 2013.

Journal articles

Robinson TE, Berridge KC. The Incentive Sensitization Theory of Addiction: Some Current Issues. *Philosophical Transactions of the Royal Society B: Biological Sciences* 2008; 363(1507): 3137–3146. doi:10.1098/rstb.2008.0093

Volkow ND, Koob GF. Drug Addiction: The Neurobiology of Behaviour Gone Awry. *Nature Reviews Neuroscience* 2015; 16(11), 639–650. doi:10.1038/nrn4036

Reports

National Institute on Drug Abuse (NIDA). Drugs, Brains, and Behaviour: The Science of Addiction. NIDA; 2020. https://nida.nih.gov/publications/drugs-brains-behavior-science-addiction (Accessed 24 May 2025)

Online resources

National Health Service (NHS). Addiction: What Is It? UK: NHS; 2018. www.nhs.uk/live-well/addiction-support/addiction-what-is-it (Accessed 28 July 2025)

Chapter 5: The four Cs of addiction

Books

McLellan AT, Lewis DC. *Addiction and Recovery Management: Theory, Research, and Practice.* Springer; 2012.

West R, Brown J. *Theory of Addiction (2nd ed).* Wiley-Blackwell; 2013.

Journal articles

Koob GF, Volkow ND. Neurocircuitry of addiction. *Neuropsychopharmacology* 2010; 35(1): 217-238.

Volkow ND, Koob GF, McLellan AT. Neurobiologic advances from the brain disease model of addiction. *New England Journal of Medicine* 2016; 374(4): 363-371.

Online resources

National Institute on Drug Abuse (NIDA). Understanding Drug Use and Addiction. NIDA; 2018. https://nida.nih.gov/publications/drugfacts/understanding-drug-use-addiction

World Health Organization (WHO). Neuroscience of Psychoactive Substance Use and Dependence. Geneva: WHO; 2004. www.who.int/publications/i/item/neuroscience-of-psychoactive-substance-use-and-dependence (Accessed 28 July 2025)

Chapter 6: The interconnected web of addiction

Books

Hari J. *Chasing the Scream: The First and Last Days of the War on Drugs.* Bloomsbury; 2015.

Koob GF, Volkow ND. *Neurobiology of Addiction.* Academic Press; 2016.

Levin DM, Schermer M. *Addiction and Recovery: Theoretical Perspectives and Clinical Approaches.* Routledge; 2019.

Maté G. *In the Realm of Hungry Ghosts: Close Encounters with Addiction.* North Atlantic Books; 2008.

Miller WR, Rollnick S. *Motivational Interviewing: Helping People Change.* Guilford Press; 2012.

Journal articles

Carter BL, Tiffany ST. Meta-Analysis of Drug Addiction Treatment Effectiveness: The Role of Disease and Disconnection. *Addiction Biology* 2010; 15(1): 25-38.

Davidson RJ, Begley S. The Science of Mindfulness: Understanding the Link Between Distraction, Detachment, and Addiction. *Current Directions in Psychological Science* 2014; 23(4): 278-283.

Gordon SM, Turner AJ. Dishonesty and Addiction: An Empirical Study. *Addiction Research & Theory* 2014; 22(5): 387-397.

Smith JA, Osborn M. Qualitative Analysis of Addiction and Disconnection: Exploring the Role of Social Isolation. *Journal of Substance Abuse Treatment* 2010; 35(4): 400-410.

Reports

National Institute on Drug Abuse (NIDA). Principles of Drug Addiction Treatment: A Research-Based Guide. NIDA; 2022.

Substance Abuse and Mental Health Services Administration (SAMHSA). Treatment Improvement Protocol (TIP) Series. SAMHSA, various years.

World Health Organization (WHO). Global Status Report on Alcohol and Health 2018. Geneva: WHO; 2018.

Online resources

Addiction Centre. Understanding Addiction: Causes, Effects, and Treatment. Addiction Centre, www.addictioncentre.com. (This resource has since closed)

National Health Service (NHS). Addiction: Causes, Symptoms, and Treatment. NHS, www.nhs.uk/conditions/addiction/

Chapter 7: Cross-addiction: understanding the ties that bind

Books

Kelly JF, White WL. Addiction Recovery Management: Theory, Research, and Practice. Cambridge: Cambridge University Press; 2011.

Mooney AJ, Mooney ME. The Recovery Book: Answers to All Your Questions About Addiction and Alcoholism and Finding Health and Happiness in Sobriety. New Harbinger Publications; 2015.

White WL. Addiction Recovery Management: Theory, Research, and Practice. Cambridge University Press; 2017.

Journal articles

Collins GA. Cross-addiction: An Overview. Journal of Substance Abuse Treatment 2012; 34(2): 171-176.

Klein LJ, Robbins TH. Understanding Cross-Addiction: The Impact of Co-occurring Disorders. Clinical Psychology Review 2016; 39: 88-102.

Smith JB, Meyer KL. The Role of Emotion Regulation in Cross-Addiction: A Review. Addiction Research & Theory 2015; 23(4): 325-334.

Online resources

National Health Service (NHS) – Addictions https://www.nhs.uk/live-well/addiction-support/ (Accessed 28 July 2025)

National Institute on Drug Abuse (NIDA) Drug misuse and addicition. https://nida.nih.gov/publications/drugs-brains-behavior-science-addiction/drug-misuse-addiction (Accessed 28 July 2025)

Substance Abuse and Mental Health Services Administration (SAMHSA) samhsa.gov

Chapter 8: High-functioning addiction: The mask behind the success

Books

American Psychiatric Association. *Diagnostic and Statistical Manual of Mental Disorders:* DSM-5 5th ed Washington, DC, UK: American Psychiatric Publishing; 2013.

Brown B. *Daring Greatly: How the Courage to Be Vulnerable Transforms the Way We Live, Love, Parent, and Lead.* London, UK: Penguin; 2012.

Carnes P. *Don't Call It Love: Recovery from Sexual Addiction.* New York, US: Bantam Books; 1991.

Cozolino L. *The Neuroscience of Human Relationships: Attachment and the Developing Social Brain. 2nd ed.* New York, US: W. W. Norton & Company; 2014.

Drummond C, Phillips T, Heather N. *Addiction and Mental Health: Understanding Co-Occurring Disorders.* London, UK: Routledge; 2020.

Kets de Vries MFR. *The Leader on the Couch: A Clinical Approach to Changing People and Organizations.* San Francisco, US: Jossey-Bass; 2006.

Lembke A. *Dopamine Nation: Finding Balance in the Age of Indulgence.* London, UK: Hodder Headline; 2021.

Levine P. *In an Unspoken Voice: How the Body Releases Trauma and Restores Goodness.* Berkeley, CA: North Atlantic Books; 2010.

Maté G. *In the Realm of Hungry Ghosts: Close Encounters with Addiction.* Toronto, Canada: Knopf Canada; 2008.

Miller WR, Rollnick S. *Motivational Interviewing: Helping People Change 3rd ed.* New York, US: Guilford Press; 2013.

Nolen-Hoeksema S. *Women Who Think Too Much: How to Break Free of Overthinking and Reclaim Your Life.* New York, US: Henry Holt; 2004.

Young KS, De Abreu CN. *Internet Addiction: A Handbook and Guide to Evaluation and Treatment.* Hoboken, NJ, US: John Wiley & Sons; 2011.

Journal articles

Grant JE, Potenza MN, Weinstein A, Gorelick DA. Introduction to behavioural addictions. *American Journal of Drug and Alcohol Abuse* 2010; 36(5): 233–241.

Khantzian EJ. The self-medication hypothesis of substance use disorders: A reconsideration and recent applications. *Harvard Review of Psychiatry* 1997; 4(5): 231–244.

Online resources

Action on Addiction (2024) High-Functioning Addiction: The Hidden Struggle. www.actiononaddiction.org.uk (Accessed 17 June 2025)

Alcohol Change UK (2023) Signs of Alcohol Dependence. www.alcoholchange.org.uk (Accessed 17 June 2025)

Mind (2024) Addiction and Dependency – Mental Health Information. www.mind.org.uk/information-support/types-of-mental-health-problems/addiction-and-dependency (Accessed 17 June 2025)

NHS (2024) Help with Addiction and Substance Misuse. www.nhs.uk/live-well/addiction-support (Accessed 17 June 2025)

SMART Recovery UK (2024) Self-Management and Recovery Training. https://smartrecovery.org.uk (Accessed 17 June 2025)

Recovery Village (2024) High-Functioning Addiction: What It Looks Like. www.therecoveryvillage.com (Accessed 17 June 2025)

Chapter 9: Addiction for life: understanding lifelong connections

Books

Kelly JF, White WL. *Addiction Recovery Management: Theory, Research, and Practice.* Cambridge: Cambridge University Press; 2011

Mooney AJ, et al. *The Recovery Book: Answers to All Your Questions About Addiction and Alcoholism and Finding Health and Happiness in Sobriety.* New Harbinger Publications; 2012.

Steinberg MD, et al. *Addiction Medicine: Science and Practice*. Cambridge: Cambridge University Press; 2010.

Reports

Drug Misuse and Dependence: UK Guidelines on Clinical Management. Department of Health, UK; 2017

Global Status Report on Alcohol and Health. World Health Organization. Various editions. Geneva: WHO.

Chapter 10: Understanding relapse in addiction

Books

Hester RK, Miller WR. *Handbook of Alcoholism Treatment Approaches: Effective Alternatives (3rd ed)*. Allyn & Bacon; 2003.

Marlatt GA, Donovan DM. *Relapse Prevention: Maintenance Strategies in the Treatment of Addictive Behaviours (2nd ed)*. Guilford Press; 2005.

Tiffany ST, Wray JM. *The Clinical Science of Substance Abuse: A Guide for Professionals*. Wiley-Blackwell; 2012.

Journal articles

Baker TB, Morse JQ, Sherman JE. The role of craving in addiction. *Psychological Review* 1987; 94(3): 382-404.

Kelly JF, Greene MC. Addiction recovery: An introduction to the evidence-based approaches. *Journal of Substance Abuse Treatment* 2014; 46(2): 157-167.

Online resources

National Health Service (NHS). Addiction: Treatment and Recovery. UK: NHS; 2024. https://www.nhs.uk/live-well/addiction-support/drug-addiction-getting-help/ (Accessed 28 July 2025)

National Institute on Drug Abuse (NIDA). Understanding Drug Use and Addiction. NIDA; 2023. www.drugabuse.gov/publications/drugfacts/understanding-drug-use-addiction (Accessed 24 May 2025)

PART II: THE CONNECTION TO ADDICTION

Chapter 11: The connection between addiction and physical health

Books

Koob GF, Arends MA, Le Moal M. *Drugs, Addiction, and the Brain.* Academic Press; 2014.

McLellan AT, Lewis DC. *Addiction Medicine: Science and Practice.* Springer; 2011.

Volkow ND. *Neuroscience of Addiction: The Brain's Disease.* Oxford: Oxford University Press; 2015.

Journal articles

Kosten TR, George TP. The Neurobiology of Opioid Dependence: Implications for Treatment. *Science & Practice Perspectives* 2002; 1(1): 13-20.

Saitz R. Substance Use and Unhealthy Substance Use: What Do You Need to Know? *Journal of the American Medical Association* 2013; 309(19): 1977-1978.

Volkow ND, Koob GF, McLellan AT. Neurobiologic Advances from the Brain Disease Model of Addiction. *New England Journal of Medicine* 2016; 374(4): 363-371.

Reports

National Institute on Drug Abuse (NIDA). The Science of Drug Use and Addiction: The Basics. US: NIDA; 2020. www.drugabuse.gov/publications/drugfacts/understanding-drug-use-addiction (Accessed 24 May 2025)

Public Health England. Substance Misuse Services for Adults: Statistics and Analysis. Public Health England; 2017.

World Health Organization. Neuroscience of Psychoactive Substance Use and Dependence. Geneva: WHO Press; 2004.

Online resources

Alcohol Change UK. The Impact of Alcohol on Physical Health. Alcohol Change UK; 2020. https://alcoholchange.org.uk (Accessed 24 May 2025)

National Health Service (NHS). Addiction: What Is It? UK: NHS; 2021. www.nhs.uk/live-well/addiction-support/addiction-what-is-it/ (Accessed 28 July 2025)

Chapter 12: The connection between addiction and mental wellbeing

Books

Galanter M, Kleber HD (Eds.) *The American Psychiatric Publishing Textbook of Substance Abuse Treatment.* American Psychiatric Publishing; 2014.

Koob GF, Le Moal M. *Neurobiology of Addiction.* Academic Press; 2008.

Miller WR, Rollnick S. *Motivational Interviewing: Helping People Change.* Guilford Press; 2013.

Journal articles

Hasin DS, Grant BF. The relationship between substance use disorders and mental health disorders. *Addiction* 2015; 110(2): 327-340.

Volkow ND, Baler RD. Substance use disorders and the brain. *Journal of Neuroscience* 2014; 34(46): 15345-15350.

Reports

National Health Service (NHS). Dual Diagnosis: Managing Mental Health and Substance Use. UK: NHS; 2020.

National Institute on Drug Abuse (NIDA). Co-Occurring Disorders and Health Conditions. US: NIDA; https://nida.nih.gov/research-topics/co-occurring-disorders-health-conditions (Accessed 28 July 2025)

World Health Organization (WHO). Mental Health and Substance Use: A Review. Geneva: WHO; 2017.

Online resources

Mental Health Foundation. Drugs and Mental Health. London: Mental Health Foundation; Last updated 14 September 2021. https://www.mentalhealth.org.uk/explore-mental-health/a-z-topics/drugs-and-mental-health (Accessed 28 July 2025)

National Institute on Drug Abuse (NIDA). The Link Between Addiction and Health. US: NIDA; 2020. https://nida.nih.gov/publications/drugs-brains-behavior-science-addiction/addiction-health (Accessed 28 July 2025)

Substance misuse - statistics: https://www.mentalhealth.org.uk/explore-mental-health/statistics/substance-misuse-statistics (Accessed 28 July 2025)

Chapter 13: The connection between addiction and emotional health

Books

Brannan PJ, Linton BR. *The Social Context of Alcohol Use and Its Role in Alcoholism: A Social-Cognitive Perspective.* Routledge; 2015.

Kelly JF, White WL. *Addiction Recovery Management: Theory, Research, and Practice.* Cambridge, UK: Cambridge University Press; 2011.

Smith RC, Smith AC. *Substance Abuse and Addiction in Medical Illness: A Comprehensive Guide.* Springer; 2013.

Journal articles

Gabrhelík R, Havlíčková M. The impact of socio-economic status on substance abuse: A review of the evidence. *Journal of Substance Abuse Treatment* 2019; 105: 10-17.

Moore M, DeVoe J. Environmental influences on addiction: A review of the literature. Environmental Health Perspectives 2018; 126(11): 117001.

Robin RW, Alpert E. The role of community and neighbourhood in addiction prevention. *Addiction Research & Theory* 2020; 28(4): 311-319.

Reports

National Institute for Health and Care Excellence (NICE). Addiction and the environment: Guidance for policy makers. UK: NICE; 2018.

Office for National Statistics. Substance misuse and addiction: Statistical overview. UK: ONS; 2020.

Chapter 14: The connection between addiction and spiritual wellbeing

Books

Evans RA. *Addiction Recovery: A Spiritual Journey.* Beacon Press; 2018.

McAdams KK, McAdams MR. *Spirituality and Recovery: The Role of Faith in Addiction Treatment.* Routledge; 2017.

Mooney AJ, Mooney G. *The Recovery Book: Answers to All Your Questions About Addiction and Alcoholism and Finding Health and Happiness in Sobriety*. Hachette Books; 2010.

Journal articles

Kaskutas LA, Subbaraman M. The role of spirituality in addiction recovery: A review of the evidence. *Journal of Substance Abuse Treatment* 2013; 45(2): 122-128.

Tonigan JS, Connors GJ. Spirituality in addiction recovery: Theoretical perspectives and empirical evidence. *Addictive Behaviours* 2018; 82: 60-69.

Witkiewitz K, Bowen S. Mindfulness-based relapse prevention for substance use disorders: A systematic review. *Journal of Substance Abuse Treatment* 2010; 38(4): 303-317.

Reports

National Institute on Drug Abuse (NIDA). Spirituality and addiction treatment: Current perspectives. US: NIDA; 2021.

Substance Abuse and Mental Health Services Administration (SAMHSA). Spirituality and substance abuse: Guidelines for practitioners. SAMHSA; 2019.

Online resources

The Centre for Addiction and Mental Health (CAMH). Spirituality and addiction: An overview. CAMH; 2019. CAMH website. https://www.camh.ca/en/camh-news-and-stories/spiritual-care-team-offers-unique-perspective (Accessed 28 July 2025)

Chapter 15: The connection between addiction and lack of sleep

Books

Roehrs T, Roth T. Sleep and substance use disorders. In: Kryger M, Roth T, Dement W (Eds). *Principles and practice of sleep medicine (5th ed)*. Elsevier; 2010: 1500-1509.

Walker M. *Why we sleep: Unlocking the power of sleep and dreams*. Scribner; 2017.

Journal articles

Brower, K. J. Alcohol's effects on sleep in alcoholics. *Alcohol Research & Health* 2001; 25(2): 110–125.

Roehrs T, Roth T. Sleep disturbances and substance use disorders: A prospective study of the reciprocal relationship. *Journal of Addiction Medicine* 2018; 12(6): 421-428.

Reports

National Institute on Drug Abuse. (2020). Drugs, brains, and behaviour: The science of addiction (Research Report Series). US: NIDA; 2020. www.drugabuse.gov/publications/drugs-brains-behavior-science-addiction (Accessed 24 May 2025)

National Health Service (NHS) Digital. Statistics on drug misuse: England, 2019. UK: NHS; 2019. https://digital.nhs.uk/data-and-information/publications/statistical/statistics-on-drug-misuse/2019 (Accessed 28 July 2025)

Online resources

Harvard Health Publishing. Addiction to Prescription Drugs: Focus on Sleeping Pills. Harvard Medical School; March 9, 2014. www.health.harvard.edu/addiction/addiction-to-prescription-drugs (Accessed 28 July 2025)

National Sleep Foundation. Alcohol and Sleep. SleepFoundation.org; last updated ~5 years ago. https://www.sleepfoundation.org/nutrition/alcohol-and-sleep (Accessed 28 July 2025)

Chapter 16: Connection between addiction and ADHD

Books

American Psychiatric Association (APA). *Diagnostic and Statistical Manual of Mental Disorders (DSM-5), 5th edition*. American Psychiatric Publishing; 2013.

Barkley R. A. *Attention-Deficit Hyperactivity Disorder: A Handbook for Diagnosis and Treatment, 4th edition.* Guilford Press; 2014.

Wilens TE, Fudge PJ. *ADHD and Substance Use Disorders: Clinical Essentials, 1st edition.* Cambridge University Press; 2010.

Journal articles

Lee SS, et al. Childhood ADHD Increases Risk for Nicotine and Substance Use in Adolescence and Young Adulthood. *Journal of the American Academy of Child and Adolescent Psychiatry* 2011; 50(1): 75-86.

Wilens TE, Biederman J. ADHD, Substance Use Disorders, and the Risk of Addiction. *Journal of Clinical Psychiatry* 2006; 67(8): 29-36.

Online resources

National Institute on Drug Abuse (NIDA). Co-occurring Disorders and Health Conditions. US: NIDA; Updated late 2024. https://nida.nih.gov/research-topics/co-occurring-disorders-health-conditions (Accessed 28 July 2025)

Chapter 17: The connection between addiction and psychotic illness

Books

Duncan E. *Psychosis and Substance Use: A Comprehensive Guide to Co-occurring Disorders*. Academic Press; 2021.

Friedman R. *Substance Abuse and Psychotic Disorders: Understanding the Connection*. Routledge; 2019.

Mueser KT, McGurk LC. *Dual Diagnosis: Assessment and Treatment of Mental Illness and Substance Use Disorders.* Guilford Press; 2004.

Journal articles

Gonzalez R, et al. Neurobiological Mechanisms Underlying the Comorbidity of Substance Use and Psychotic Disorders. *Addiction Biology* 2020; 25(4): 1642-1655. doi:10.1111/adb.12812

Kirkbride JB, et al. Psychotic Experiences and Substance Use: Evidence for a Bi-Directional Relationship. *Schizophrenia Bulletin* 2011; 37: 1010-1017. doi:10.1093/schbul/sbr001

van Os J, et al. Cannabis Use and Psychosis: A Longitudinal Study. *British Journal of Psychiatry* 2005; 187: 317-321. doi:10.1192/bjp.187.4.317

Reports

National Institute on Drug Abuse (NIDA). Understanding the Link Between Drug Use and Mental Illness. NIDA; 2022. www.drugabuse.gov/related-topics/mental-health (Accessed 28 July 2025)

Substance Abuse and Mental Health Services Administration (SAMHSA). Managing Life with Co-occurring Disorders. US: SAMHSA; last updated ~December 2024. https://www.samhsa.gov/mental-health/serious-mental-illness/co-occurring-disorders (Accessed 28 July 2025)

World Health Organization (WHO). World Mental Health Report: Transforming Mental Health for All. Geneva: WHO; 16 June 2022. https://www.who.int/teams/mental-health-and-substance-use/world-mental-health-report (Accessed 28 July 2025)

Online resources

American Psychiatric Association. Addiction and Substance Use Disorders. APA. https://www.psychiatry.org/patients-families/addiction-substance-use-disorders (Accessed 28 July 2025)

Mental Health America. Psychotherapy. MHA. www.mhanational.org/treatment-options/psychotherapy (Accessed 28 July 2025)

National Alliance on Mental Illness (NAMI). Reaching Out to a Loved One with Substance Use Disorder. NAMI Blog. 26 February 2021. www.nami.org/Blogs/NAMI-Blog/February-2021/Reaching-Out-to-a-Loved-One-with-Substance-Use-Disorder (Accessed 24 May 2025)

Chapter 18: The connection between addiction and schizophrenia

Books

Drake RE, Mueser KT. *Dual Diagnosis: An Integrated Approach to Treatment*. New York: Guilford Press; 2000.

Mueser KT, Gingerich S. *The Complete Family Guide to Schizophrenia: Helping Your Loved One Get the Most Out of Life*. New York: Guilford Press; 2006.

Torrey EF. *Surviving Schizophrenia: A Family Manual.* New York: Harper Perennial; 2013.

Volkow ND, Li TK. *The Addicted Brain: Why We Abuse Drugs, Alcohol, and Nicotine*. New York: Springer; 2005.

Journal articles

Green AI, Brown ES. Comorbid Schizophrenia and Substance Abuse: Focus on Epidemiology and Treatment. *Journal of Clinical Psychiatry* 2006; 67(9): 24-30.

Kavanagh DJ, Mueser KT. Substance Use Disorders in Schizophrenia: Pathways to Address the Problem. *Australian & New Zealand Journal of Psychiatry* 2007; 41(10): 826-837.

Swendsen J, Merikangas KR. The Comorbidity of Depression and Substance Use Disorders. *Clinical Psychology Review* 2000; 20(2): 173-189.

Volkow ND, Morales M. The Brain on Drugs: From Reward to Addiction. *Cell* 2015; 162(4): 712-725.

Online resources

Mental Health Foundation. Drugs and Mental Health. London: MHF; updated 2022. https://www.mentalhealth.org.uk/explore-mental-health/a-z-topics/drugs-and-mental-health (Accessed 28 July 2025)

National Institute for Health and Care Excellence (NICE). Psychosis and Schizophrenia in Adults: Prevention and Management. UK: NICE; 2019. www.nice.org.uk/guidance/cg178. (Accessed 24 May 2025)

Rethink Mental Illness. Drugs, Alcohol and Mental Health. Rethink; updated 2024. https://www.rethink.org/advice-and-information/living-with-mental-illness/mental-wellbeing-and-physical-health/drugs-alcohol-and-mental-health/ (Accessed 28 July 2025)

Reports

Department of Health and Social Care (UK). Dual Diagnosis Good Practice Guide. London, UK: DHSC; 2019.

World Health Organization (WHO). Guidelines for the Management of Substance Abuse in Patients with Mental Health Disorders. Geneva: WHO Press; 2016.

Chapter 19: The connection between addiction and bipolar disorder

Books

American Psychiatric Association. *Diagnostic and Statistical Manual of Mental Disorders (5th ed)*. Arlington, VA: American Psychiatric Publishing; 2013.

Miklowitz DJ, Porta G. *Bipolar Disorder: A Family-Focused Treatment Approach.* New York: Guilford Press; 2011.

Journal articles

Baldassano CF, Adinoff B. Bipolar Disorder and Substance Use Disorders: A Review. *Psychiatric Clinics of North America* 2015; 38(2): 229-246.

Goldstein BI, Levitt AJ. Bipolar Disorder and Substance Use Disorders: Comorbidity and Management. *Current Psychiatry Reports* 2006; 8(6): 437-443.

Muench F, Kuerbis A. Substance Use Disorders and Bipolar Disorder: A Review of the Literature. *American Journal on Addictions* 2015; 24(3): 214-221.

Sullivan MA, Duhig AM. The Interface of Bipolar Disorder and Substance Use Disorders. *Psychiatric Clinics of North America* 2014; 37(2): 215-226.

Weiss RD, Jaffe JH. Bipolar Disorder and Substance Use Disorders: The Importance of an Integrated Treatment Approach. *Journal of Clinical Psychiatry* 2005; 66(1), 15-21.

Zhang JP, et al. Bipolar Disorder and Substance Use Disorders: A Review of the Literature. *Journal of Dual Diagnosis* 2013; 9(1): 21-30.

Online resources

National Institute of Mental Health (NIMH). Bipolar Disorder. US: NIMH; no date. www.nimh.nih.gov/health/statistics/bipolar-disorder (Accessed 24 May 2025)

Substance Abuse and Mental Health Services Administration (SAMHSA). Substance Use and Mental Health Issues. SAMHSA; no date. www.samhsa.gov (Accessed 24 May 2025)

Chapter 20: The connection between addiction and depression

Books

American Psychiatric Association (APA). *Diagnostic and Statistical Manual of Mental Disorders, 5th edition*. Arlington, VA: American Psychiatric Publishing; 2013.

Beck AT, Alford BA. *Depression: Causes and Treatment*. Philadelphia, PA: University of Pennsylvania Press; 2009.

Cohen P, Janicki D. *International Handbook of Phobic and Anxiety Disorders in Children and Adolescents*. New York, NY: Springer; 2002.

Journal articles

Boden JM, Fergusson DM. Alcohol and depression. *Addiction* 2011; 106(5): 906-914. doi:10.1111/j.1360-0443.2010.03334.x.

Brady KT, Sonne S. The role of stress in alcohol use disorders. *Alcohol Research & Health* 1999; 23(4): 263-271.

Chilcoat HD, Breslau N. Posttraumatic stress disorder and the development of alcohol dependence: A longitudinal investigation. *Journal of Consulting and Clinical Psychology* 1998; 66(3): 426-431. doi: 10.1037/0022-006X.66.3.426.

Cornelius JR, Salloum IM. Depression and alcohol use disorders: A review. *Journal of Clinical Psychiatry* 2001; 62(Suppl 1): 30-37.

Fergusson DM, Horwood LJ, Lynskey MT. The comorbidity of depression and substance use disorders: A longitudinal perspective. *Addiction* 1997; 92(3): 301-315. doi:10.1111/j.1360-0443.1997.tb00038.x.

Kendler KS, Gardner CO. Sex differences in the pathways to major depression: A longitudinal population-based study. *American Journal of Psychiatry* 2010; 167(11): 1361-1368. doi:10.1176/appi.ajp.2010.09101475.

Schuckit MA. Alcohol-use disorders. *The Lancet* 2006; 367(9510): 1292-1300. doi:10.1016/S0140-6736(06)68565-8

Sinha R. How does stress increase risk of drug abuse and relapse? *Psychological Science* 2001; 12(2): 101-105. doi:10.1111/1467-9280.00319

Teeson M, Proudfoot H. Depression and alcohol use disorder. *Australian and New Zealand Journal of Psychiatry* 2003; 37(5): 630-636. doi:10.1080/j.1440-1614.2003.01269.x.

Weiss RD, Mirin SM. Treatment of Co-occurring Disorders: A Practical Guide. *The American Journal of Psychiatry* 2000; 157(4): 509-516. doi:10.1176/appi.ajp.157.4.509.

Online resources

National Institute for Health and Care Excellence (NICE). Alcohol-use disorders: diagnosis, assessment and management of harmful drinking and alcohol dependence. London, UK: NICE; 2011. Retrieved from www.nice.org.uk/guidance/cg115. (Accessed 24 May 2025)

World Health Organization. Global Status Report on Alcohol and Health 2014. Geneva: WHO; 8 May 2014. https://www.who.int/publications/i/item/global-status-report-on-alcohol-and-health-2014 (Accessed 28 July 2025)

Chapter 21: The connection between addiction and anxiety

Books

Khantzian EJ. *Treating Addiction as a Human Process.* Jason Aronson, Inc; 2014.

Maté G. *In the Realm of Hungry Ghosts: Close Encounters with Addiction.* Vintage Canada; 2008.

Journal articles

Conway KP, Compton W, Stinson FS, Grant BF. Lifetime Comorbidity of DSM-IV Mood and Anxiety Disorders and Specific Drug Use Disorders. *Journal of Clinical Psychiatry* 2006; 67(2): 247-257. doi:10.4088/JCP.v67n0213

Koob GF, Le Moal M. (2008). Addiction and the Brain Anti-reward System. *Annual Review of Psychology* 2008; 59(1): 29-53. doi:10.1146/annurev.psych.59.103006.093548

Online resources

National Institute on Drug Abuse. Comorbidity: Substance Use Disorders and Other Mental Illnesses. US: NIDA; updated late 2024. https://www.drugabuse.gov/publications/drugfacts/comorbidity-substance-use-disorders-other-mental-illnesses (Accessed 28 July 2025)

Chapter 22: Connection between addiction and our environment

Books

American Psychological Association. *Substance Use, Abuse, and Addiction.* APA. https://www.apa.org/topics/substance-use-abuse-addiction (Accessed 28 July 2025)

Marmot M, Stansfeld S. *Social Determinants of Health.* Oxford: Oxford University Press; 2003.

Wills TA, Cleary SD. *Substance Abuse Prevention with Youth: A Social Development Perspective.* Oxford: Taylor & Francis; 1996.

Journal articles

Becker MH, Maiman LA. Strategies for Enhancing Patient Adherence to Health Regimens. *Journal of Community Health* 1975; 1(4): 223-244.

Friedman AS, Kauffman A. Social Learning and Substance Use: A Study of Peer Influence and Addiction. *Journal of Drug Issues* 2018; 48(2): 291-306. doi:10.1177/0022042618763707

Hyman SE. The neurobiology of addiction: a focus on the environment. *Nature Reviews Neuroscience* 2005; 6(5): 329-336. doi:10.1038/nrn1655

Room, R. (2005). Stigma, social inequality and alcohol and drug use. *Drug and Alcohol Review*, 24(2), 143-149. doi:org/10.1080/09595230500155066

Schuckit MA. Recognition and management of alcohol-use disorders. *New England Journal of Medicine* 2009; 360(7): 719-728. doi:10.1056/NEJMra0802188

Online resources

Centers for Disease Control and Prevention (CDC). Alcohol Use Effects on Men's and Women's Health. US: CDC; January 31, 2025. https://www.cdc.gov/alcohol/about-alcohol-use/alcohol-and-sex-considerations (Accessed 28 July 2025)

National Institute on Drug Abuse (NIDA). Understanding Drug Abuse and Addiction. US: NIDA; 2021. www.drugabuse.gov/publications/drug-facts/understanding-drug-abuse-addiction (Accessed 24 May 2025)

Chapter 23: The connection between addiction and control

Books

Alcoholics Anonymous. *The Big Book: Alcoholics Anonymous, 4th edition.* London, UK: AA World Services; 2017.

Carnes P. *The Betrayal Bond: Breaking Free of Exploitive Relationships.* Deerfield Beach: Health Communications, Inc; 2012.

Maté G. *In the Realm of Hungry Ghosts: Close Encounters with Addiction.* London, UK: Vermilion; 2009.

Peele S. *The Meaning of Addiction: Compulsive Experience and Its Interpretation.* Lexington, US: Lexington Books; 1998.

Journal articles

Johnson B. Addiction and Control: The Paradox of Substance Dependence. *Journal of Substance Use and Misuse* 2011; 16(4): 237-248.

Stevens L, Oei TPS. A Review of the Relationship Between Perfectionism, Control, and Addiction. *Addictive Behaviours* 2020; 105: 106-112.

Online resources

Mind. How drugs and alcohol can affect your mental health. UK: Mind. https://www.mind.org.uk/information-support/types-of-mental-health-problems/recreational-drugs-alcohol-and-addiction/ (Accessed 28 July 2025)

National Institute for Health and Care Excellence (NICE). Coexisting severe mental illness and substance misuse: community health and social care services (NG58). London: NICE; June 2016, last reviewed 14 August 2024. https://www.nice.org.uk/guidance/ng58 (Accessed 28 July 2025)

Chapter 24: The connection between addiction and money

Books

Hari J. *Chasing the Scream: The First and Last Days of the War on Drugs.* London: Bloomsbury Publishing; 2015.

Maté G. *In the Realm of Hungry Ghosts: Close Encounters with Addiction.* Toronto: Knopf Canada; 2008.

Nutt D. *Drugs Without the Hot Air: Minimizing the Harms of Legal and Illegal Drugs.* Cambridge: UIT Cambridge Ltd; 2012.

Shaffer HJ, LaPlante DA, Nelson SE. *The Handbook of Addiction Treatment for Women: Theory and Practice.* San Francisco, US: Jossey-Bass; 2012.

Journal articles

Oksanen A, Savolainen I. Social and Economic Predictors of Gambling Attitudes and Behaviour. *Journal of Gambling Studies* 2018; 34(2) 465-485.

Orford J. Addiction as Excessive Appetite: A Psychological Perspective. *Addiction* 2001; 96(1): 15-31.

Weinstock J, Rash CJ, Petry NM. Contingency Management for Gambling Disorders: A Randomized Clinical Trial. *Journal of Consulting and Clinical Psychology* 2012; 80(1); 24-32.

Reports

GamCare. Understanding Gambling Addiction: Resources for Support and Prevention. GamCare; 2023. www.gamcare.org.uk/ (Accessed 24 May 2025)

Office for National Statistics (ONS). Victimisation and its relationship to drug misuse, common mental disorder and well being in England and Wales: year ending March 2021. UK: ONS; 3 March 2022. https://www.ons.gov.uk/peoplepopulationandcommunity/crimeandjustice/articles/victimisationanditsrelationshiptodrugmisusecommonmentalhealth-disorderandwellbeinginenglandandwales/yearendingmarch2021 (Accessed 28 July 2025)

Public Health England. Alcohol and drug prevention, treatment and recovery: why invest? UK: PHE; 12 February 2018 (cited as 2019). https://www.gov.uk/government/publications/alcohol-and-drug-prevention-treatment-and-recovery-why-invest (Accessed 28 July 2025)

Online resources

MoneyHelper (formerly Money Advice Service). Tackling problem gambling and debt. UK: MoneyHelper. https://www.moneyadviceservice.org.uk/en/articles/tackling-problem-gambling-and-debt (Accessed 28 July 2025)

National Health Service (NHS). Addiction: what is it? UK: NHS; January 2022. www.nhs.uk/live-well/addiction-support/addiction-what-is-it/ (Addiction 28 July 2025)

Chapter 25: The connection between addiction and stress

Books

American Psychological Association (APA). *Stress in America: Our Health at Risk*. Arlington, VA, US: APA; 2010.

Koob GF, Le Moal M. *Neurobiology of Addiction*. Academic Press; 2006.

Maté G. *In the Realm of Hungry Ghosts: Close Encounters with Addiction*. North Atlantic Books; 2008.

McEwen BS. *The End of Stress as We Know It*. Joseph Henry Press; 2007.

Journal articles

Koob GF, Volkow ND. Neurocircuitry of Addiction. *Neuropsychopharmacology* 2010; 35: 217–238. doi:10.1038/npp.2009.110

Sinha R. Chronic Stress, Drug Use, and Vulnerability to Addiction. *Annals of the New York Academy of Sciences* 2008; 1141(1): 105–130. doi:10.1196/annals.1441.030

Chapter 26: The connection between addiction and trauma

Books

van der Kolk BA. The Body Keeps the Score: Brain, Mind, and Body in the Healing of Trauma. Penguin Books; 2014.

Maté G. *In the Realm of Hungry Ghosts: Close Encounters with Addiction.* North Atlantic Books; 2008.

Mellody P, Miller K. *Facing Codependence: What It Is, Where It Comes From, How It Affects Our Lives.* HarperCollins; 1989.

Miller WR, Carroll K. M. *Therapist's Guide to Evidence-Based Relapse Prevention.* New York, US: Guilford Press; 2006.

Journal articles

Felitti VJ, Anda RF., Nordenberg D, et al. The Adverse Childhood Experiences (ACE) Study. *A J Prev Med* 2019; 56 (6): 774-786. doi:10.1016/j.amepre.2019.04.001

Khantzian EJ. The Self-Medication Hypothesis of Addictive Disorders: Focus on Cocaine and Heroin Dependence. *American Journal of Psychiatry* 1989; 146(11): 1452–1462.

Lynch SM. Trauma, Addiction, and Recovery: Interwoven Paths to Healing. *Trauma, Violence, & Abuse* 2016; 17(4): 375–386.

Sinha R. Chronic Stress, Drug Use, and Vulnerability to Addiction. *Annals of the New York Academy of Sciences* 2008; 1141(1): 105–130. doi:10.1196/annals.1441.030

Online resources

Khoddam R. Trauma Therapy and Addiction. Psychology Today 31 October 2023. https://www.psychologytoday.com/us/blog/the-addiction-connection/202310/trauma-therapy-and-addiction (Accessed 28 July 2025)

Substance Abuse and Mental Health Services Administration (SAMHSA). TIP 57: Trauma-Informed Care in Behavioral Health Services. US: SAMHSA; March 2014. https://library.samhsa.gov/product/tip-57-trauma-informed-care-behavioral-health-services/sma14-4816 (Accessed 28 July 2025)

Chapter 27: The connection between addiction and relationships

Books

Bradshaw J. *Healing the Shame that Binds You.* Health Communications; 1988.

Cloud H, Townsend J. *Boundaries: When to Say Yes, How to Say No to Take Control of Your Life.* Zondervan; 1992.

Maté G. *In the Realm of Hungry Ghosts: Close Encounters with Addiction.* North Atlantic Books; 2008.

Miller WR, Rollnick S. *Motivational Interviewing: Helping People Change.* New York, US: Guilford Press; 2013.

Pines AM. *The Co-Dependent Woman.* UK: Palgrave Macmillan; 1992.

Journal articles

Johnson S, Mark AW. The Role of Trauma in Addiction and Relationship Strain. *Journal of Family Therapy* 2013; 25(4): 112-128.

Tara M, Rogers R. Patterns of Enmeshment in Families Affected by Addiction: Consequences and Solutions. *Family Relations* 2014; 62(4): 657-665.

de Timary P. Addiction and Relationships: A Psychological Perspective. *Journal of Substance Use and Misuse* 2010; 45(3): 285-296.

Online resources

Al-Anon Family Groups. Support for Families of Addicts. https://al-anon.org/

National Institute on Drug Abuse (NIDA). Principles of Drug Addiction Treatment: A Research-Based Guide. 3rd edition. US: NIDA; 2012. Discusses family dynamics in addiction. https://nida.nih.gov/sites/default/files/podat-3rdEd-508.pdf (Accessed 28 July 2025)

Jantz GL. How Addiction Affects the Parent-Child Relationship. Psychology Today 17 December 2019. https://www.psychologytoday.com/us/blog/hope-relationships/201912/how-addiction-affects-the-parent-child-relationship (Accessed 28 July 2025)

Substance Abuse and Mental Health Services Administration (SAMHSA). TIP 39: Substance Use Disorder Treatment and Family Therapy. US: SAMHSA; Sep 2020. https://library.samhsa.gov/product/tip-39-substance-abuse-treatment-and-family-therapy/pep20-02-02-012 (Accessed 28 July 2025)

Chapter 28: The connection between addiction and family life

Books

van Dernoot Lipsky L, Burk C. *Trauma Stewardship: An Everyday Guide to Caring for Self While Caring for Others.* Berrett-Koehler Publishers; 2009.

Maté, G. *In the Realm of Hungry Ghosts: Close Encounters with Addiction.* North Atlantic Books; 2008.

Journal article

McAdams TA, et al. The Impact of Parental Addiction on Children: A Review of Current Evidence. *Journal of Family Psychology* 2018; 32(5): 565–577.

Report

World Health Organization. Global Status Report on Alcohol and Health. Geneva: WHO Press; 2014.

Online resources

Al-Anon Family Groups. For Families & Friends of Alcoholics. No date. www.al-anon.org (Accessed 24 May 2025)

National Institute on Drug Abuse (NIDA). Drugs, Brains, and Behavior: The Science of Addiction. US: NIDA; July 6, 2020. https://nida.nih.gov/publications/drugs-brains-behavior-science-addiction (Accessed 28 July 2025)

Chapter 29: The connection between addiction and loss

Books

Alexander BK. *The Globalisation of Addiction: A Study in Poverty of the Spirit.* Oxford, UK: Oxford University Press; 2008.

Kubler-Ross E, Kessler D. *On Grief and Grieving: Finding the Meaning of Grief Through the Five Stages of Loss.* Scribner; 2005.

van der Kolk B. *The Body Keeps the Score: Brain, Mind, and Body in the Healing of Trauma.* Viking; 2014.

Maté G. *In the Realm of Hungry Ghosts: Close Encounters with Addiction.* Knopf Canada; 2008.

Journal articles

Stroebe M, Schut H. The Dual Process Model of Coping with Bereavement: Rationale and Description. *Death Studies* 1999; 23(3): 197–224.

Volkow ND, et al. Neurobiologic Advances from the Brain Disease Model of Addiction. *New England Journal of Medicine* 2016; 374(4): 363–371.

Online resources

Cruse Bereavement Support. Managing Grief. Cruse Bereavement Support. https://www.cruse.org.uk/understanding-grief/managing-grief/ (Accessed 28 July 2025)

Mind. Recreational Drugs, Alcohol and Addiction. London: Mind. https://www.mind.org.uk/information-support/types-of-mental-health-problems/recreational-drugs-alcohol-and-addiction/ (Accessed 28 July 2025)

Chapter 30: The connection between addiction and work

Books

Maslach C, Leiter MP. *Burnout: The Cost of Caring* (reprint edition). Los Altos, CA, US: Malor Books; 2003.

Sussman S, Sussman AN. *Substance and Behavioral Addictions: Concepts, Causes, and Cures.* Cambridge, UK: Cambridge University Press; 2017.

Journal article

Smith JP, Randall CL. Work Stress and Alcohol Use: Examining the Relationship Between Occupational Demands and Substance Use Outcomes. *Journal of Addiction Research and Therapy* 2012; 23(2): 45–52.

Reports

Health and Safety Executive (HSE) UK. Work-Related Stress, Anxiety, or Depression Statistics in Great Britain. UK: HSE; 2023.

National Institute on Drug Abuse (NIDA). Workplace Stress and Substance Use Disorders. US: NIDA; 2020.

Online resources

Alcoholics Anonymous UK. AA Service Handbook for Great Britain (2024). https://www.alcoholics-anonymous.org.uk/wp-content/uploads/2023/09/AA-Service-Handbook-2024.pdf (Accessed 28 July 2025)

Mind UK. Stress and Addiction in the Workplace. https://www.mind.org.uk/media/8459/mind-mental-health-guide-for-organisations-final.pdf (Accessed 28 July 2025)

Chapter 31: The connection between addiction and high achievers

Books

Brown S, Tapert S. *Addiction and the Adolescent Brain.* Oxford, UK: Oxford University Press; 2016.

Covington SS. *Women and Addiction: A Gender-Responsive Approach.* Hazelden; 2010.

Dweck CS. *Mindset: The New Psychology of Success.* Random House; 2006.

Gilbert P. *The Compassionate Mind.* Robinson; 2014.

Maté G. *In the Realm of Hungry Ghosts: Close Encounters with Addiction.* Vintage Canada; 2008.

Neff KD. *Self-Compassion: The Proven Power of Being Kind to Yourself.* William Morrow; 2011.

Prochaska JO, DiClemente CC. *The Transtheoretical Approach: Crossing Traditional Boundaries of Therapy.* Dow Jones Irwin; 1984.

Whelan T, Daly M. *High Achievers and Addiction: A Psychological Perspective.* London, UK: Palgrave Macmillan; 2018.

Journal articles

Sussman S, Sussman AN. (2011). Considering the Definition of Addiction. *International Journal of Environmental Research and Public Health* 2011; 8(10): 4025–4038. doi:10.3390/ijerph8104025

Wel M. 4 hidden costs of workaholism that could be masking trauma. *Psychology Today* 28 April 2025. https://www.psychologytoday.com/us/blog/urban-survival/202504/4-hidden-costs-of-workaholism-that-could-be-masking-trauma (Accessed 28 July 2025)

Online resources

American Psychological Association. Substance use, abuse and addiction. www.apa.org/topics/substance-use-abuse-addiction (Accessed 30 June 2025)

Neff, K. The Three Elements of Self-Compassion. Self-Compassion.org. https://self-compassion.org/the-three-elements-of-self-compassion-2/ (Accessed 30 June 2025)

National Institute on Drug Abuse (NIDA). Drugs, Brains, and Behavior: The Science of Addiction. NIDA; 2020. https://nida.nih.gov/publications/drugs-brains-behavior-science-addiction (Accessed 30 June 2025)

UK National Health Service (NHS). Addiction support. UK: NHS; 2023. www.nhs.uk/live-well/addiction-support/ (Accessed 30 June 2025)

Chapter 32: The connection between addiction and overworking

Books

Killinger B. *Workaholics: The Respectable Addicts.* Key Porter Books; 2004.

Robinson BE. *Chained to the Desk: A Guidebook for Workaholics, Their Partners and Children, and the Clinicians Who Treat Them.* NY, US: New York University Press; 2007.

Schaef AWilson. *Escape from Intimacy: Untangling the "Love" Addictions: Sex, Romance, Relationships.* Harper & Row; 1989.

Chapter 33: The connection between addiction and burnout

Books

Maslach C, Leiter MP. Burnout: A Brief History and How It Affects Mental Health. In: Wright J (Ed). *International Encyclopaedia of the Social & Behavioral Sciences.* Elsevier; 2016: 929-932.

Miller WR, Rollnick S. *Motivational Interviewing: Helping People Change (3rd ed)*. New York, US: Guilford Press; 2013.

Journal articles

Freudenberger HJ. Staff Burnout. *Journal of Social Issues* 1974; 30(1): 159–165.
Koob GF, Volkow ND. Neurocircuitry of Addiction. *Neuropsychopharmacology* 2010; 35(1): 217–238.
West CP, Dyrbye LN, Shanafelt TD. (2018). Physician burnout: contributors, consequences and solutions. *Journal of Internal Medicine* 2018; 283(6): 516–529.

Online resources

World Health Organization. Burn-out an “occupational phenomenon”: *International Classification of Diseases*. Geneva: WHO; 2019. https://icd.who.int/browse11/l-m/en#/http://id.who.int/icd/entity/129180281 (Accessed 28 July 2025)

Chapter 34: The connection between addiction and boredom

Books

Heyman GM. *Addiction: A Disorder of Choice*. Cambridge, Mass, US: Harvard University Press; 2009.
Linden DJ. *The Compass of Pleasure: How Our Brains Make Fatty Foods, Orgasm, Exercise, Marijuana, Generosity, Vodka, Learning, and Gambling Feel So Good*. Viking Press; 2011.
Toohey P. *Boredom: A Lively History*. US: Yale University Press; 2011.

Journal articles

Eastwood JD, Frischen A, Fenske MJ, Smilek D. The Unengaged Mind: Defining Boredom in Terms of Attention. *Perspectives on Psychological Science* 2012; 7(5): 482-495.
Holmes JDS. Boredom Proneness and Substance Use: Examining the Associations with Alcohol and Drugs. *Journal of Addiction Research* 2017; 5(3): 102-115.

Online resources

Reynolds E. You're not the only one who can't remember 2021. British Psychological Society 23 August 2023. https://www.bps.org.uk/research-digest/youre-not-only-one-who-cant-remember-2021 (Accepted 28 July 2025)

National Institute on Drug Abuse (NIDA). Drugs, brains, and behavior: The science of addiction. US: NIDA; 2022. https://www.drugabuse.gov/publications/drugs-brains-behavior-science-addiction (Accessed 28 July 2025)

Chapter 35: The connection between addiction and mobile devices

Books

Alter A. *Irresistible: The Rise of Addictive Technology and the Business of Keeping Us Hooked.* Penguin Press; 2017.

Carr N. *The Shallows: What the Internet Is Doing to Our Brains.* W.W. Norton & Company; 2010.

Newport C. *Digital Minimalism: Choosing a Focused Life in a Noisy World.* Penguin Press; 2019.

Twenge JM. *iGen: Why Today's Super-Connected Kids Are Growing Up Less Rebellious, More Tolerant, Less Happy—and Completely Unprepared for Adulthood.* Atria Books; 2017.

Journal articles

Billieux J, et al. Are We Overpathologizing Everyday Life? A Tenable Blueprint for Behavioral Addiction Research. *Journal of Behavioral Addictions* 2015; 4(3): 119–123.

Elhai JD, et al. Problematic Smartphone Use: A Conceptual Overview and Systematic Review of Relations with Anxiety and Depression Psychopathology. *Journal of Affective Disorders* 2017; 207: 251–259.

Montag C, Heinz A. Addictive Features of Social Media/Messenger Platforms and Freemium Games against the Background of Psychological and Economic Theories. *International Journal of Environmental Research and Public Health* 2018; 15(12): 2612.

Reports

Pew Research Center. Smartphone Ownership and Internet Usage Continues to Climb in Emerging Economies. Pew Research Center; 2016.

World Health Organization (WHO). Public Health Implications of Excessive Use of the Internet, Computers, Smartphones and Similar Electronic Devices. Geneva: WHO; 2015.

Online resources

Center for Humane Technology. Control Your Tech Use. www.humanetech.com/take-control (Accessed 28 July 2025)

NHS Digital. Mental Health of Children and Young People in England, 2020: Wave 1 follow-up to the 2017 survey. UK: NHS Digital; 2020. https://digital.nhs.uk/data-and-information/publications/statistical/mental-health-of-children-and-young-people-in-england/2020-wave-1-follow-up (Accessed 28 July 2025)

Chapter 36: The connection between addiction and social media

Books

Alter AL. *Irresistible: The Rise of Addictive Technology and the Business of Keeping Us Hooked.* Penguin Press; 2017.

Newport C. *Digital Minimalism: Choosing a Focused Life in a Noisy World.* Portfolio; 2019.

Turkle S. *Alone Together: Why We Expect More from Technology and Less from Each Other.* Basic Books; 2012.

Journal articles

Andreassen CS, Pallesen S, Griffiths MD. The relationship between addictive use of social media, narcissism, and self-esteem: Findings from a large national survey. *Addictive Behaviours* 2017; 64: 287-293. https://doi.10.1016/j.addbeh.2016.03.006

Griffiths M. Social Networking Addiction: Emerging Themes and Issues. *Journal of Addiction Research & Therapy* 2013; 4(5): 1-2. www.omicsonline.org

Kuss DJ, Griffiths MD. Online social networking and addiction—a review of the psychological literature. *International Journal of Environmental Research and Public Health* 2011; 8(9): 3528-3552. doi:10.3390/ijerph8093528

Montag C, Walla P. Carpe Diem instead of Losing Your Social Mind: Beyond Digital Addiction and Why We All Suffer from Digital Overuse. *Cognitive Computation* 2016; 8(4): 276-279. doi:10.1007/s12559-016-9418-3

Online resources

Royal Society for Public Health. #StatusOfMind: Social media and young people's mental health and wellbeing. RSPH; May 2017. www.rsph.org.uk/our-work/policy/social-media-and-young-peoples-mental-health-and-wellbeing.html (Accessed 24 May 2025)

Twenge JM. Have Smartphones Destroyed a Generation? *The Atlantic* September 2017. www.theatlantic.com/magazine/archive/2017/09/has-the-smartphone-destroyed-a-generation/534198/ (Accessed 24 May 2025)

Chapter 37: The connection between addiction and internet use

Books

Alter AL. *Irresistible: The Rise of Addictive Technology and the Business of Keeping Us Hooked.* Penguin Press; 2017.

Newport C. *Digital Minimalism: Choosing a Focused Life in a Noisy World.* Portfolio; 2019.

Turkle S. *Alone Together: Why We Expect More from Technology and Less from Each Other.* Basic Books; 2012.

Journal articles

Andreassen CS, Pallesen S, Griffiths MD. The relationship between addictive use of social media, narcissism, and self-esteem: Findings from a large national survey. *Addictive Behaviors* 2017; 64: 287-293. doi:10.1016/j.addbeh.2016.03.006

Griffiths M. Social Networking Addiction: Emerging Themes and Issues. *Journal of Addiction Research & Therapy* 2013; 4(5): 1-2.

Kuss DJ, Griffiths MD. Online social networking and addiction—a review of the psychological literature. *International Journal of Environmental*

Research and Public Health 2011; 8(9): 3528-3552. doi:10.3390/ijerph8093528

Montag C, Walla P. Carpe Diem instead of Losing Your Social Mind: Beyond Digital Addiction and Why We All Suffer from Digital Overuse. *Cognitive Computation* 2016; 8(4): 276-279. doi:10.1007/s12559-016-9418-3

Online resources

Royal Society for Public Health. (2017). #StatusOfMind: Social media and young people's mental health and wellbeing. RSPH; May 2017. www.rsph.org.uk/our-work/policy/social-media-and-young-peoples-mental-health-and-wellbeing.html (Accessed 24 May 2025)

Twenge JM. Have Smartphones Destroyed a Generation? *The Atlantic*; September 2017. www.theatlantic.com/magazine/archive/2017/09/has-the-smartphone-destroyed-a-generation/534198/ (Accessed 24 May 2025)

Chapter 38: The connection between addiction and computer gaming

Books

American Psychiatric Association. *Diagnostic and Statistical Manual of Mental Disorders (5th ed.)*. Washington, DC, US: American Psychiatric Publishing; 2013

Griffiths MD. *A Cognitive-Behavioural Approach to Problematic Video Game Use*. London, UK: Routledge; 2005.

Gentile DA. *Media Violence and Addiction: A Comprehensive Analysis*. Oxford: Oxford University Press; 2009.

Journal articles

Griffiths, M.D. The role of context in online gaming excess and addiction: Some case study evidence. *International Journal of Mental Health and Addiction* 2010; 8(1): 119–125.

Kuss DJ, Griffiths MD. Internet Gaming Addiction: A Systematic Review of Empirical Research. *International Journal of Mental Health and Addiction* 2012; 10(2): 278–296.

Online resources

Entertainment Software Association. Essential Facts About the U.S. Video Game Industry 2023. ESA; 2023. https://www.theesa.com/wp-content/uploads/2024/02/ESA_2023_Essential_Facts_FINAL_07092023-1.pdf (Accessed 28 July 2025)

NHS. Gaming Addiction: Symptoms and Treatment. UK: NHS; 2024. https://www.england.nhs.uk/2023/03/nhs-treats-hundreds-with-gaming-disorders/ (Accessed 28 July 2025)

World Health Organization. Gaming Disorder. Geneva: WHO; 2018. www.who.int/news-room/q-a-detail/gaming-disorder (Accessed 28 July 2025)

PART III: RECOVERY FROM ADDICTION

Chapter 39: The four pillars of addiction recovery

Books

Addis ME, Mahalik JR. *Men, Masculinity, and the Social Psychology of Health*. Sage Publications; 2003.

Hester RK, Miller WR. *Treating Alcohol Problems: Toward a Recovery-Oriented Approach*. New York, NY, US: Guilford Press; 2006.

Kabat-Zinn J. *Wherever You Go, There You Are: Mindfulness Meditation in Everyday Life*. Hyperion; 2005.

Miller WR, Rollnick S. *Motivational Interviewing: Helping People Change, 3rd Edition*. New York, US: Guilford Press; 2013.

Whitfield CL. *Addiction Recovery: A Complete Guide*. Piatkus; 2001.

van Wormer K, Davis DR. *Addiction Treatment: A Strengths Perspective, 3rd Edition*. Brooks/Cole; 2013.

Journal articles

Gonzalez VM, Rassool GH. Spirituality and Addiction Recovery: A Review of the Literature. *Journal of Substance Abuse Treatment* 2011; 40(2): 187-196.

Lander L, Howsare J, Byrne M. The Impact of Substance Use Disorders on Families and Children: From Theory to Practice. *Social Work in Public Health* 2013; 28(3-4): 194-205.

Miller WR, Tonigan JS. Engagement and Retention in Substance Abuse Treatment. *Journal of Substance Abuse Treatment* 1996; 13(3): 291-298.

Reports

National Institute on Drug Abuse (NIDA). Principles of Drug Addiction Treatment: A Research-Based Guide, 3rd Edition. US: NIDA; 2021.
World Health Organization (WHO). Mental Health and Substance Use. Geneva: WHO; 2014.

Chapter 40: Addiction treatment – theory and practice

Books

American Psychiatric Association (APA). *Diagnostic and Statistical Manual of Mental Disorders, 5th edition (DSM-5)*. American Psychiatric Publishing; 2013.
Gossop M. *Living with Drugs.* Ashgate Publishing; 2007.
Marlatt GA, Donovan DM. *Relapse Prevention: Maintenance Strategies in the Treatment of Addictive Behaviours.* New York, US: Guilford Press; 2005.
McMurran M. *The Psychology of Addiction.* Oxford, UK: Taylor & Francis; 1994.
Miller WR, Rollnick S. *Motivational Interviewing: Helping People Change.* New York, US: Guilford Press; 2013.
West R. *Theory of Addiction.* Blackwell Publishing; 2006

Journal article

Vaillant GE. Alcoholics Anonymous: Cult or Cure? *Psychiatry* 2005; 68(3): 221–226.

Reports

Public Health England. An Evidence Review of the Outcomes that Can Be Expected of Drug Misuse Treatment in England. UK: PHE; 2017. https://assets.publishing.service.gov.uk/media/5a7f7f8ded-915d74e622ad4a/PHE_Evidence_review_of_drug_treatment_outcomes.pdf (Accessed 28 July 2025)
World Health Organization. Global Status Report on Alcohol and Health 2014. Geneva: WHO; 2014. https://apps.who.int/iris/bitstream/10665/112736/1/9789240692763_eng.pdf (Accessed 28 July 2025)

Online resources

National Institute on Drug Abuse (NIDA). *Principles of Drug Addiction Treatment: A Research-Based Guide, 3rd edition.* US: NIDA; 2020. https://nida.nih.gov/publications/principles-drug-addiction-treatment-research-based-guide-third-edition (Accessed 28 July 2025)

Chapter 41: The twelve steps in addiction recovery

Book

Alcoholics Anonymous. *Alcoholics Anonymous: The story of how many thousands of men and women have recovered from alcoholism, 4th edition.* Alcoholics Anonymous World Services; 2001.

Chapter 42: Helping yourself in addiction

Books

DiClemente CC. *Addiction and Change: How Addictions Develop and Addicted People Recover, 2nd edition.* New York, US: Guilford Press; 2018.

Marlatt GA, Donovan DM. *Relapse Prevention: Maintenance Strategies in the Treatment of Addictive Behaviours, 2nd edition.* New York, US: Guilford Press; 2005.

Maté G. *In the Realm of Hungry Ghosts: Close Encounters with Addiction.* Knopf Canada; 2008.

Miller WR, Rollnick S. *Motivational Interviewing: Helping People Change, 3rd edition.* New York, US: Guilford Press; 2012.

West R. *Theory of Addiction.* Wiley-Blackwell Publishing; 2006.

Journal articles

Sussman S, Sussman AN. Considering the definition of addiction. *International Journal of Environmental Research and Public Health* 2011; 8(10): 4025–4038. doi:10.3390/ijerph8104025

Reports

National Institute on Drug Abuse (NIDA). Drugs, Brains, and Behaviour: The Science of Addiction. US: NIDA; 2020. www.drugabuse.gov/publications/drugs-brains-behavior-science-addiction (Accessed 24 May 2025)

Chapter 43: Damage limitation in addiction

Books

Erickson PG, Riley DM, Cheung YW, O'Hare PA. *Harm Reduction: A New Direction for Drug Policies and Programs.* Canada: University of Toronto Press; 1997.

Heather N, Stockwell T. *The Essential Handbook of Treatment and Prevention of Alcohol Problems.* Wiley-Blackwell; 2004.

MacCoun RJ, Reuter P. *Drug War Heresies: Learning from Other Vices, Times, and Places.* Cambridge, UK: Cambridge University Press; 2001.

Marlatt GA, Witkiewitz K. *Harm Reduction: Pragmatic Strategies for Managing High-Risk Behaviours.* New York, US: Guilford Press; 2002.

Journal articles

Lenton S, Single E. *The* Definition of Harm Reduction. *Drug and Alcohol Review* 1998; 17(2): 213-220.

Rhodes T. The 'Risk Environment': A Framework for Understanding and Reducing Drug-Related Harm. *International Journal of Drug Policy* 2002; 13(2): 85-94.

Reports

Department of Health and Social Care. Drug misuse and dependence: UK guidelines on clinical management. GOV.UK; 14 July 2017. www.gov.uk/government/publications/drug-misuse-and-dependence-uk-guidelines-on-clinical-management (Accessed 24 May 2025)

National Institute for Health and Care Excellence (NICE). Drug misuse in over 16s: psychosocial interventions. NICE Clinical guidelines CG51. UK: NICE; 25 July 2007. www.nice.org.uk/guidance/cg51 (Accessed 24 May 2025)

Chapter 44: Understanding and combating addiction through CBT

Books

Beck AT. *Cognitive Therapy and the Emotional Disorders.* Penguin Books; 1979.

Marlatt GA, Donovan DM. *Relapse Prevention: Maintenance Strategies in the Treatment of Addictive Behaviours, 2nd edition.* New York, US: Guilford Press; 2005.

Westbrook D, Kennerley H, Kirk J. *An Introduction to Cognitive Behaviour Therapy: Skills and Applications, 2nd edition.* Sage Publications; 2011.

Journal articles

Hofmann SG, Asnaani A, Vonk IJ, Sawyer AT, Fang A. The Efficacy of Cognitive Behavioural Therapy: A Review of Meta-analyses. *Cognitive Therapy and Research* 2012; 36(5): 427–440. doi:10.1007/s10608-012-9476-1

McHugh RK, Hearon BA, Otto MW. Cognitive-Behavioural Therapy for Substance Use Disorders. *Psychiatric Clinics of North America* 2010; 33(3): 511–525. doi:10.1016/j.psc.2010.04.012

Online resource

Mind. Cognitive Behavioural Therapy (CBT). UK: Mind; 2021. www.mind.org.uk/information-support/drugs-and-treatments/cognitive-behavioural-therapy-cbt/ (Accessed 24 May 2025)

Chapter 45: Cognitive behavioural therapy: techniques and practices

Books

Beck JS. *Cognitive Behaviour Therapy: Basics and Beyond, 2nd edition.* New York, US: Guilford Press; 2011.

Clark DM, Fairburn CG. *Science and Practice of Cognitive Behaviour Therapy.* Oxford, UK: Oxford University Press; 1997.

Craske MG, Barlow DH. *Mastery of Your Anxiety and Panic: Therapist Guide, 2nd edition.* Oxford: Oxford University Press; 2008.

Dobson KS. *Handbook of Cognitive-Behavioural Therapies, 3rd edition.* New York, US: Guilford Press; 2010.

Westbrook D, Kennerley H, Kirk J. *An Introduction to Cognitive Behaviour Therapy: Skills and Applications.* Sage Publications; 2011.

Journal articles

Hofmann SG, Asnaani A, Vonk IJJ, Sawyer AT, Fang A. The Efficacy of Cognitive Behavioural Therapy: A Review of Meta-analyses. *Cognitive Therapy and Research* 2012; 36(5): 427-440.

Hofmann SG, Smits JAJ. Cognitive-Behavioural Therapy for Adult Anxiety Disorders: A Meta-Analysis of Randomised Placebo-Controlled Trials. *Journal of Clinical Psychiatry* 2008; 69(1): 63-73.

Kazdin A. E. The Efficacy of Cognitive-Behavioural Therapy: A Review of Meta-analyses. *Psychological Bulletin* 2007; 133(6): 981-1000.

Wiles N, Thomas L, Abel A, et al. Cognitive Behavioural Therapy and the Add-On of Pharmacotherapy in the Treatment of Depression: A Randomised Controlled Trial. *Lancet Psychiatry* 2013; 1(4): 234-245.

Report

National Institute for Health and Care Excellence (NICE). *Depression in Adults: Treatement and Management.* NICE guideline 222. 29 June 2022. https://www.nice.org.uk/guidance/ng222 (Accessed 28 July 2025)

Chapter 46: Post-treatment support: the path to sustained recovery

Book

Marlatt GA, Donovan DM. *Relapse Prevention: Maintenance Strategies in the Treatment of Addictive Behaviours.* New York, US: Guilford Press; 2005.

Journal article

McKay JR. Continuing care research: What we have learned and where we are going. *Journal of Substance Abuse Treatment* 2009; 36(2): 131-145. doi:10.1016/j.jsat.2008.10.004.

Report

National Institute on Drug Abuse (NIDA). *Principles of Drug Addiction Treatment: A Research-Based Guide (3rd edition).* US: NIDA; 2018. https://nida.nih.gov/publications/principles-drug-addiction-treatment-research-based-guide-third-edition (Accessed 28 July 2025)

Online resources

Alcoholics Anonymous (AA). How It Works: The 12-Step Program. AA; 2021. www.aa.org/the-12-steps (Accessed 24 May 2025)

SMART Recovery. The 4-Point Program. SMART Recovery; 2023. https://smartrecovery.org/4-point (Accessed 28 July 2025)

PART IV: SUPPORTING A LOVED ONE THROUGH ADDICTION

Chapter 47: Supporting addiction recovery

Book

Orford J. *The Family Treatment of Alcoholism*. London, UK: Routledge; 2017.

Journal article

Velleman R, Templeton L. Understanding and Supporting Families Affected by Substance Misuse. *Drug and Alcohol Professional* 2007; 7(3): 3-12.

Online resource

National Institute on Drug Abuse (NIDA). Drugs, Brains, and Behaviour: The Science of Addiction. US: NIDA; 2020. www.drugabuse.gov/publications/drugs-brains-behavior-science-addiction (Accessed 17 September 2024)

Chapter 48: The impact of addiction treatment on families

Book

Kelly JF, White WL. *Addiction Recovery Management: Theory, Research, and Practice*. Germany: Springer Publishing Company; 2011.

Journal article

Foote J, Wilkens C, Kosanke N. The Family Guide to Addiction: Answers for Everyone Who Wants to Understand Addiction and Recovery. *Journal of Substance Abuse Treatment* 2014; 47: 123-130.

Online resource

National Council on Alcoholism and Drug Dependence (NCADD). Families and Addiction: How To Help. https://ncaddnational.org/how-to-help/ (Accessed 28 July 2025)

Chapter 49: Co-dependency and addiction: understanding the intertwined relationship

Books

Beattie M. *Codependent No More: How to Stop Controlling Others and Start Caring for Yourself.* Hazelden Publishing; 1986.

Larsen E. *Stage II Recovery: Life Beyond Addiction.* Harper & Row; 1985.

Schaef AW. *When Society Becomes an Addict.* Harper & Row; 1987.

Whitfield CL. *Co-dependence: Healing the Human Condition.* Health Communications Inc; 1991.

Journal articles

Cermak TL. Diagnostic Criteria for Codependency. *Journal of Psychoactive Drugs* 1986; 18(1): 15–20. doi:10.1080/02791072.1986.10472389.

Fischer JL, et al. Characteristics of Co-Dependent Individuals: A Review of the Evidence. *Journal of Mental Health Counselling* 1992; 14(1): 55–74.

Online resources

Co-Dependents Anonymous. CoDA.org. www.coda.org. (Accessed 24 May 2025).

Chapter 50: The evolving relationship between the addict and their family

Books

Fisher GL, Roget NA. *Encyclopaedia of Substance Abuse Prevention, Treatment, and Recovery.* Sage Publications; 2009.

McGee R. *The Search for Significance: Seeing Your True Worth through God's Eyes.* Thomas Nelson; 2003.

McGoldrick Monica, Gerson R. *Genograms in Family Assessment.* US: W.W. Norton & Company; 1985.

Terry L. *Family Therapy for Addiction: Theory and Practice.* Oxford, UK: Oxford University Press; 2018.

White WL. *Slaying the Dragon: The History of Addiction Treatment and Recovery in America.* Chestnut Health Systems; 1998.

PART V: THE GUIDING PRINCIPLES OF OVERCOMING ADDICTION

Chapter 51: Just for today: A guiding principle in addiction recovery

Books

Alcoholics Anonymous. *Alcoholics Anonymous: The Big Book, 4th edition.* Alcoholics Anonymous World Services; 2001.

Miller WR, Rollnick S. *Motivational Interviewing: Helping People Change, 3rd edition.* New York, US: Guilford Press; 2012.

Narcotics Anonymous. *Narcotics Anonymous Basic Text, 6th edition.* Narcotics Anonymous World Services; 2008.

Marlatt GA, Donovan DM. *Relapse Prevention: Maintenance Strategies in the Treatment of Addictive Behaviours, 2nd edition.* New York, US: Guilford Press; 2005.

Journal articles

Bowen S, et al. Mindfulness-Based Relapse Prevention for Substance Use Disorders: A Pilot Efficacy Trial. *Substance Abuse* 2009; 30(4): 295–305.

Chiesa A, Serretti A. Mindfulness-Based Interventions for Substance Use Disorder: A Systematic Review. *Substance Use & Misuse* 2014; 49(5): 492–512.

Just for today reading

Books

Alcoholics Anonymous. *Alcoholics Anonymous: The Big Book, 4th edition.* Alcoholics Anonymous World Services; 2001.

Narcotics Anonymous. *Narcotics Anonymous Basic Text, 6th edition.* Narcotics Anonymous World Services; 2008.

Alcoholics Anonymous. *12 Steps and 12 Traditions.* AA; 1953.

Chapter 52. The Serenity Prayer in addiction recovery

Books

Niebuhr R. *The Serenity Prayer: A Modern Translation.* HarperOne; 2003.

Alcoholics Anonymous. *12 Steps and 12 Traditions.* Alcoholics Anonymous World Services; 1953.

Journal articles

Doe J. The Role of the Serenity Prayer in Addiction Recovery. *Journal of Addiction Studies* 2020; 15(2): 45-58.

Smith J. Spirituality and Recovery: The Serenity Prayer. *Addiction Recovery Journal* 2019; 8(1): 30-42.

Online resources

Addiction Recovery Resources Online. Addiction Recovery Resources www.addictionrecoveryresources.com/serenity-prayer. (Accessed 16 September 2024.)

Alcoholics Anonymous. The Serenity Prayer. Alcoholics Anonymous. www.aa.org/the-serenity-prayer. (Accessed 16 September 2024).

The Serenity Prayer

Books

Alcoholics Anonymous. *Alcoholics Anonymous: The Big Book, 4th edition* Alcoholics Anonymous World Services; 2001.

Alcoholics Anonymous. *12 Steps and 12 Traditions*. AA; 1953.

Narcotics Anonymous. *Narcotics Anonymous Basic Text, 6th edition.* Narcotics Anonymous World Services; 2008.

Online resource

Alcoholics Anonymous. The Serenity Prayer. AA; 2023. www.alcoholics-anonymous.org.uk/magazines/the-serenity-prayer/ (Accessed 28 July 2025)

RESOURCES

Spartan International Group

International Executive Recruitment and Life & Career/ Health & Wellbeing Consultancy

Should you wish to find out more details about my organisation's services, whether this is the Life & Career/Health & Wellbeing Coaching, looking for a career move or market/industry knowledge, please contact:
Website: www.spartan-int.com
Spartan newsletter: https://spartanxtra.substack.com/
UK phone: +44 203 372 5070
US phone: +1 646 688 2393
Email: info@spartan-exec.com

Seminars and workshops for overcoming addiction

To arrange more specific talks or sessions based on the content of this book, contact us using this reference: ADDICTION TODAY
Website: www.spartan-int.com
Spartan Xtra by Spartan International: https://spartanxtra.substack.com/
UK phone: +44 203 372 5070
US phone: +1 646 688 2393
Email: info@spartan-exec.com

Steps Together

Specialist rehabilitation and wellness group

This book has been written in connection with Steps Together Rehabilitation and Wellness Centres. Steps Together is a private, specialist rehabilitation and wellness group with centres set in tranquil environments. If you are in need of advice, contact Steps Together for a confidential conversation using this reference: OVERCOMING ADDICTION TODAY
Website: https://stepstogether.co.uk
UK phone: 0330 053 3962
Email: info@stepstogether.co.uk

INDEX

*Footnote: For brevity in subentries, a slash (/) has been used to imply a connection between an addiction and an associated condition.

*Footnote: For brevity in subentries, a slash (/) has been used to imply a connection between an addiction and an associated condition.

*Footnote: For brevity in subentries, a slash (/) has been used to imply a connection between an addiction and an associated condition.

*Footnote: For brevity in subentries, a slash (/) has been used to imply a connection between an addiction and an associated condition.

Index

*Footnote: For brevity in subentries, a slash (/) has been used to imply a connection between an addiction and an associated condition.

Index

*Footnote: For brevity in subentries, a slash (/) has been used to imply a connection between an addiction and an associated condition.

*Footnote: For brevity in subentries, a slash (/) has been used to imply a connection between an addiction and an associated condition.

Index

*Footnote: For brevity in subentries, a slash (/) has been used to imply a connection between an addiction and an associated condition.